$\frac{q}{l}$

All patient testimonies are real and names have been abbreviated for privacy. No testimonial was paid for in any way. No editing has occurred in the testimonials so any typos are there for authenticity. Dr. Spages has over 2500 testimonials.

"A fascinating overview of how the body works ... and how chiropractic can help achieve wellness naturally. Dr. Jonathan Spages manages to mix personal experience and professional expertise to create a volume that is both interesting and informative. The chapter on "Why Did I Get Sick" should be "must reading" for all people interested in living a better, healthier life."

Terry A. Rondberg, DC,
President, The Chiropractic Journal; Founder and CEO,
The World Chiropractic Alliance, author of *"Chiropractic First."*

"Dr. Spages stepped to the plate and hit a Health Care Home Run. If you ever wondered why so many people are turning to Chiropractic care for health solutions, this book tells us why. A must read for the health conscious."

Michael Boyd
Executive Director, Living Wellness

"Nothing is more important than our health so why wait until your body breaks down and when it does it may be so severe that surgery is needed. Dr. Spages gives us a way to gain high energy and vitality something we all want so follow your innermost thoughts that you are feeling right know that says yes I want to feel GREAT and read 'The Wellness Approach' and make that commitment to your health—now"

Dr. Louis Leonardi
Doctor and author of the book *"Pre Surgical Care"*

i

"Dr. Jonathan Spages is dedicated and passionate about bringing the latest and best information to his patients. This book is no different. He discusses the fundamentals that are missing in average Americans life. He gives an easy to follow guide to getting healthy again, the way our bodies were designed. At a time when the health of our nation gets worse and worse, this books timing is perfect."

Drs. Tom and Stephanie Chaney
Owners of Living Health Chiropractic and Functional Medicine,
www.MyLivingHealth.com

"The information Dr. Spages shares simplifies many questions and answers as to the true cause of disease, anyone who values their health will enjoy this informative and inspiring book."

Dr. James Galgano D.C.
Burlington Chiropractic, NJ, Director, Pierce Results Seminars

"When I first met Dr. Jonathan Spages, I had been chronically ill for years. I caught every cold and was effected by every seasonal allergy there was. I was fed up with every Doctor and medication I had tried since no one could diagnose me and no pill could cure me. I had tried it all and none of it worked! I was ready to go under the knife to repair a deviated septum; a procedure I was assured would stop my chronic illnesses. The only problem was I knew others who had the same operation but were still getting sick. It was then that Dr. Spages came into my life and applied the chiropractic method known as Pierce to my problems. Over a short period of time I began to heal. Now, it's a rare event to catch a cold and the debilitating symptoms of Allergies are a thing of the past. I never did get that operation. I never needed it. If your story sounds like mine then the wisdom that's in this book could be exactly what you've been searching for."

Jay Trelease
Radio and Television Broadcaster

"I have been coming here a few months, and while my health concerns are not completely gone, I have noticed a connection! I've been amazed at

how the results of my thermal scans so perfectly depict my physical health. I am amazed at how loose I feel after my adjustments and look forward to better and better health (and more well days!)"

C. R.

Actual Patient

"Since I've started getting adjusted I've noticed a tremendous difference in the way that I've been sleeping! I can actually go through an entire night without waking up or being disturbed. My mind seems to be more focused in the results of getting adjusted. I used to have the worst menstrual cramps, and I would take Vicodin to soothe the pain but now ever since my adjustments there's no need for Vicodin. Thank You!!!"

O. T.

Actual Patient

"Ever since I started chiropractic therapy with Doctor Spages I don't get headaches anymore, I feel like I could run a marathon and nothing will hurt, that's how good I feel. I would proudly recommend anybody to Dr. Spages. Dr. Spages tells you and changes you whole prospective on chiropractic. He informs you of everything that goes around you body. Chiropractic therapy helps you heel your body without any medications and makes it heel natural."

J. G.

Actual Patient

"Before starting the Chiropractic Care I could not lift my right arm from the bed after sleeping all night. I would take my left hand and lift the right arm up and bring it over to my side in order to get out of bed every morning. Now, after one week of therapy, I can lift my right arm and shoulder and get out of bed in a normal fashion, plus reach over and touch the alarm clock with the same right hand."

D. D.

Actual Patient

"Thank you Dr. Spages. I work with young children (pre school teacher) I had much difficulty sitting on the floor and getting off the floor. Back pains were a part of my daily schedule. Since I started coming for my weekly adjustments I can play on the floor with my students. My back pains have stopped and I have great days. I have changed my eating habits and have regular exercise. Dr. Spages' talks have been informative, interesting and just real good."

Y. S.

Actual Patient

"I am feeling more energetic since I have completed the first set of testimonials. I am more flexible. My balance has improved. Less menstrual cramps. I am a lot calmer. I enjoy walking again."

M. D.

Actual Patient

"When I first started coming here my lower back, neck, headaches, and shooting pain in my neck up to my head. I have been coming here for 7 months now and I haven't had any shooting pain in my neck, headaches don't happen as much, decreased pain in my lower back and neck. I would like to thank Dr. Spages and his staff for taking such great care of me. I would recommend everyone to be under the care of Dr. Spages."

C. L.

Actual Patient

"My blood pressure was always elevated about 200/100 now it is in a normal range. I had a lot of back and leg pain much improved. I am taking a lot less pain medication. Some days I don't need any at all."

J. H.

Actual Patient

"I walked into the office having headaches everyday, if not everyday. As I started to get adjusted and doing the correct exercises for myself, I have experienced a lot less headaches. Now they have lessened to maybe

a couple a month. I also use to get allergies every fall. This is my first fall under Dr. Spages and have had NO sign of the "fall" allergies at all."

H. Y.
Actual Patient

"Oh my God!! Three weeks ago I was in the emergency room because I could not speak. My throat was swollen on the inside. The emergency room Dr. gave me Lavaquin for throat infection. Dr. Spages said it was from my spine, not infection. Two days ago I came back with severe pain. I did the neck exercise Dr. Spages showed me. Two days later the pain went from a 10 to a 2 without that expensive medication. This was absolutely amazing. Thanks Dr. Spages"

D. O.
Actual Patient

"I came here about a year and a half ago after being in a coma. I had water retention on my legs, and other medications from my doctors didn't stop the pain, including eating certain vegetables. I was told I had a year and half to live and I over came that. After coming to see Dr. Spages things changed in my life. I started to feel much better, I felt like my previous Dr. didn't care about my health like Dr. Spages. Thanks to him I'm a better person."

A.R.
Actual Patient

"I have suffered with low back issues for several years. After surgery 4 years ago, I continued to have discomfort, pain and stiffness. Physical therapy helped but did not bring me to a high ensured level of functionality. Once beginning treatments with Dr. Spages, much of my stiffness was relieved and I have been able to a high level of relief and motion in my lower back increasing my ability to function at a better level."

J. Y.
Actual Patient

"One of the biggest improvements I've noticed is a decrease in allergic reactions. For the first time in over 10 years I didn't need to take any

allergy medications. I owe this to my chiropractic care. I would expect my allergies to go down even more in the next couple of years."

F. E.
Actual Patient

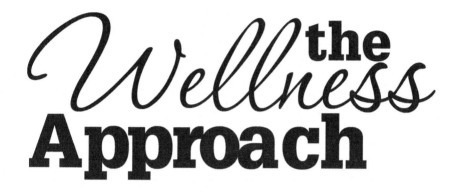

the Wellness Approach

the **SECRETS** of **HEALTH**
YOUR DOCTOR IS **AFRAID** TO TELL YOU

DR. JONATHAN B. SPAGES

NEW YORK

the *Wellness* Approach
the **SECRETS** of **HEALTH**
YOUR DOCTOR IS **AFRAID** TO TELL YOU

by **DR. JONATHAN B. SPAGES**

ISBN 978-1-60037-830-0 (paperback)
Library of Congress Control Number: 2010931989

Published by:

MORGAN JAMES PUBLISHING
The Entrepreneurial Publisher
5 Penn Plaza, 23rd Floor
New York City, New York 10001
(212) 655-5470 Office
(516) 908-4496 Fax
www.MorganJamesPublishing.com

Cover Design by:
Rachel Lopez
Rachel@r2cdesign.com

Interior Design by:
Bonnie Bushman
bbushman@bresnan.net

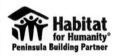
Habitat for Humanity®
Peninsula Building Partner

In an effort to support local communities, raise awareness and funds, Morgan James Publishing donates one percent of all book sales for the life of each book to Habitat for Humanity.
Get involved today, visit
www.HelpHabitatForHumanity.org.

Dedication

With All My Love—*For Mom*

Contents

Introduction

Have you ever wondered why we get sick? Is it the pollution around us? Is it something in our blood? What is it that makes us ill? Did you know that thousands of cells work together in our body to create many functions that enable us to walk, talk, breathe and enjoy life? But, most often when the body functions as it should, we tend to take it for granted. It is interesting to note that a child born sick will do everything to get healthy and when a child born healthy somehow does everything wrong to become sick. Health is taken for granted!

Nature shows us how we can live healthy and productive lives, if we only just follow its rules, the same rules which have worked for thousands of years. I believe in treating the *whole* body. That's what I'm going to teach you in this book—how to be healthy and more importantly live healthy lives.

We have become lazy as a society, where living in a bathroom connected to the internet will keep us alive for a while. You could make money, order food, get a drycleaner, order clothes, and get educated. This is an obvious way to not get the proper movement and exercise.

Indeed, our bodies have a lot to be grateful to nature for; we are incredible machines and we have been created with built-in healing

1

functions. Break your arm, for instance, and it will eventually mend. No matter what medicine can do, the body is the best healer we have. Now if only stress and our modern lifestyle wouldn't get in the way...why do some people smoke for years and not get sick and others smoke for a short time and get stricken with sickness and breathing problems.

We will look at stress because it acts like a blockage in the body that prevents our own internal healing system from working effectively.

The good news is that there is a special science which helps discover and remove that blockage, using a coordinated system for finding and fixing a primary cause of sickness and disease. Imagine a military strategy that is the major effort to finding that reason you haven't got well. Looking at the major problem where things start can make a great impact.

Stress impacts the entire body, from the bones in the spine to the nerves that run underneath, to the organs that those nerves link to.

I believe in giving the body the tools it needs to help itself. Traditional medicine tries to take things away and remove organs. It isn't about adding more life or more health; it's about taking it away. What do I mean by that? Well, it is not always best to give you pills, carry out invasive examinations or perform surgery—all of which add foreign stresses or chemicals to the body.

Instead, imagine how amazing it would be if you remove anything that shouldn't be there—to remove the causes of stress within the body that impact on its ability to heal itself.

Let's look for the underlying cause of any problem you may have; that's important, because finding the cause will ensure that the problem won't recur. Alternatively, you could take some pills and simply be treated for your symptoms. Would you rather pop pills to treat your allergies, or rid yourself of them altogether?

In this book, I am going to give you a lot of insight into strategies of treating the entire body. I'm going to explain to you with easy-to-follow analogies exactly what I do and what it stands for. I'm also going to talk in detail about the particular method that I practice— the *Pierce Results System*, unheard of since so few doctors' practice this method.

When I first started in healthcare, I couldn't understand why people had to have so many treatments before they could start becoming healthy again. Don't get me wrong; the fact that they were getting better from illnesses that had plagued them for years and years was miraculous. Still, I didn't think they should have to wait until after 20, 30 or even 60 treatments before they started to feel an effect; perhaps I was impatient. I wanted to see immediate results.

I think that's why I fell in love with the Pierce system as soon as I found it. It really is that incredible!

Throughout the book you'll find real testimonials from real people telling you, in their own words, just how they got helped. And I think you'll agree that when you hear their stories of how they can move again, breathe comfortably again, even cry again— all things they couldn't do before the treatment. I love each week in my practice getting numbers of testimonials or failed surgeries and patients who have exhausted what they thought were all their options, and they get helped.

Wellness is important to me. That's why I want to share with you my understanding of nature; I believe a great deal of illness and disease are being caused by modern-day living. The technology that we use, and the lifestyle changes that have come with it, have brought incredible advances but we pay the price as well—in the form of various diseases and illnesses.

Nature tells us so much about how we should be treating our bodies—and yet we constantly ignore it. We ignore the fact that our bodies are made for moving and exercise, and we sit on our butts all day; we pretend we eat well, but we stuff ourselves full of chocolate and processed food. We pump so many chemicals into the air that it's no wonder more and more people are having difficulty breathing.

For years we knew how to eat well; we'd eat what was available in nature when and where we found it. We would always be on the move; that gave us exercise. We weren't exposed to "modern day technology"—pesticides, chemicals, processed foods. We were healthier then—and in my view, we can get there again. After all, life can truly be enjoyed when you're in good health; if you feel fit and energetic, you can live the life that wouldn't be available when you're sick and suffering.

Compare that with feeling sick, whether you're suffering from a cold, an allergy, pain, or lack of movement—everything stops, doesn't it? Our bodies grind to a halt; all we can think about is our illness. We can't concentrate on anything else.

In this book, I'm going to tell you what you can do to take control of your health. You'll learn the steps you can take to get rid of stress—and its resulting consequences on the body.

I am going to talk about how to tackle your allergies; I'm going to discuss why you may be having problems losing weight and how you can boost your immune system to help you be cold-free.

As a father, I also have strong opinions on childbirth and raising children; you can bet I have a view on vaccines too. I have found that there is a lot of bad information out there that should be exposed.

Studies show that patients could possibly have an immune system 400% stronger than cancer patients, without taking drugs. So, congratulations! Thank you for being ready to understand more about health and living a better quality of life. You picked up this book because you thought I might have something to tell you, something new, exciting, and different than what you currently know, and I sure do!

As you apply the ideas in this book you will see huge differences in your health. I took the guesswork out of it, so you can achieve your goals quicker. Follow the simple steps in this book and use them in your daily life. Please send feedback too info@thewellnessapproachbook.com. You will see how easy it is. Let's get started on your adventure to health and success!

Chapter 1

How Does the Body Work?

To understand the importance of being fit and healthy, and how it can contribute towards the body's health, you must first understand how the body works.

Before you were as big as you are, you started as two little cells. Thank your mom and dad. As development happened, your first organs developed. Those original organs were the brain and spinal cord. It is interesting to note that the only organ fully covered in stone are your brain and spinal cord.

So first, know that all the information that you need for your body to actually work is coming from your brain. It is your brain that tells your heart to pump blood and oxygen around your body; it tells your limbs to move and your throat to swallow, as well as a hundred other orders every second or so.

How do the messages get to the right areas? Simply put, information comes from the brain and goes down a spinal cord and into all these different nerves underneath.

These nerves branch out like the branches of a tree. In fact, the nervous system of our body is similar to an upside-down tree. Information travels from the roots along the branches of the tree and to the fruit at the end of those branches; when it comes to the human body, simply substitute the fruit for bodily organs!

To start a book out this way I wanted to get back to basics. Our health care is so confusing that we stepped away from the basic fundamentals. I have discovered after seeing so many cases that the hardest problem sometimes, have some of the easiest solutions.

So looking back everything starts with the brain, the nerves, and spine. When giving lectures to patients they often think that the heart controls everything, it doesn't. However, the heart is still very important. The brain and spinal cord control everything in your body. I am at a disadvantage. This book will never win against the things you know. 120 pages or so is competing against 3000 or more hours of drug ads, commercials you will see at the end of a year. If at times I repeat an idea I know I am, to illustrate a point not to be a nagging grandmother.

Chapter 2

The Role of Stress in the Body

What is stress? Why, regardless of where we live or what we do, are we surrounded by it? Think about it, even people who live in areas where you would think there is no stress because of the beautiful weather and an amazing lifestyle that they too are subject to stress. Stress has the ability to creep up on the richest people's doorsteps and the poorest people's doorsteps, equally.

There are three types of stress commonly known: physical, chemical, and emotional. A lot of research has gone into exactly that topic; after all, if we know what contributes to ill health, we'd do everything we could to prevent it from taking hold in the first place wouldn't we? The next step of researchers was to work out why people were getting sick in the first place.

So what did they do? Doctors started looking for this thing they called 'Dis –ease'—a lack of ease in the body; nowadays we know this as stress. (It makes sense doesn't it? What else is stress but a lack of ease in the body?)

It's the one thing doctors of all branches of medicine, be it dentistry, medicine or any other branch, agree on—that 'dis-ease', or stress, is the cause of all sickness. Stress on the feet—*bunions*.

Stress on the teeth—*cavities*. Stress on the heart—*heart attacks*. Stress on the mind—mental *illness*. Stress on the spine—*nerve and organ problems.*

That's because even though our bodies are designed to cure themselves, stress gets in the way. Stress causes lack of ease in the body, which in turn interferes with the body's ability to heal itself or to run smoothly, which in turn causes sickness. Remember the upside-down tree?

So 'stress', all doctors agree, is what makes people sick!

Different health disciplines just vary in the way that they treat it.

Chapter 3

Fine Tuning the Body

So, let's expose the three types of stress. One of the more objective diagnostic tools is the very common and still very effective radiograph, also known as *x-ray*. Patients may complain for a short period of time about a particular problem they have, however, their x-ray clearly illustrates the problem has been there much longer, sometimes 10-15 years prior to their complaints.

Despite all stresses possibly creating this, let's first look at physical stress. So, let's think back to the beginning of our first days outside the womb. It is hard to believe, but our first common stress may have been a passionate and willing doctor pulling us out of our mothers, to lead us to our first breath of air. This pulling may have lead to a stress directly at the tip of the neck. Mothers and those responsible for the delivery of your first day don't check for this physical stress. Let's continue looking at our physical stress may have an effect.

Next, we learn to crawl and lift our heads. Some studies show that we fall up to 1500 times just learning how to walk.

We want to know why a person *gets* sick. We know that the underlying cause of any illness is in the brain and spinal cord—so what do we do? We actually go and fix that. We fine-tune the body!

Even the father of medicine, Hippocrates, told us to look at the spine as the cause of many diseases—and that was as long ago as 360BC!

You already know that the reason why the bones in the spine are so important is that they are right next to the spinal cord. If you put a pressure at the spinal cord a lot of things can happen. Even if there is 1% pressure on the spinal cord, it's enough to cause problems in the health of a person.

Let's take an example:

Picture if you can, your brain. Marvelous things, brains! Now, if you can, imagine that your brain has a 100% life in it— they check whether a person's living or dead through their brain activity, after all!

Luckily yours is 100% alive; now you just need that life or energy to get to the rest of your body. How this would happen— namely, is that it passes down the spinal cord, into your nerves and into the organs that they connect to. Great!

Except… sometimes not all of that life or energy makes it to where it is supposed to go.

Remember that stress earlier in this book? As we grow up and live our lives nowadays, we are subject to a lot of stress. Some of it comes from normal 'wear and tear' on the body, while in later years it can also come from the choices that we make.

But even in growing up, our bodies have to deal with stress. They say that within the first two years, a baby falls approximately 1,500 times. That's a lot of jarring on the bones!

Now our bodies are amazing things and they're created to solve a lot of problems themselves; hurt your feet walking, for instance, and a blister forms to protect the damaged skin underneath. And that's just one tiny example.

Our body corrects a lot of those faults; it can't quite correct all of them on its own. It needs help. After all of those falls, there will still be some problems within the spine. So what do we do? We add to it!

The child grows up and starts playing with other kids in the rough and tumble of the play ground; sometimes they fall, sometimes they hurt themselves. Each one of these falls adds to the problems caused by earlier injuries, causing little problems and misalignments in the spine.

Now, if you can imagine that there are 24 bones in the spine and one of those bones goes slightly out of place - only very slightly, but it's enough to cause nerve interference.

Let's say it stops the communication from the brain to the body by about 10%; remember the nerves in the spinal cord have a very important purpose. They are there to pass information along from the brain to the rest of the body; if they are impeded in any way, not all of that information can get through.

Well, if we had a 100% life in our brain, and a bone being misaligned causes 10% interference, how much of it would get to the body? It's not a trick question! That's right, 90%.

Very simply put, how can the body be healthy when working at only 90%?

Now let's say that another injury occurs—maybe a fall on the ice, or when you're playing sports—and another 10% goes out.

Well, your body is now only 80% efficient and organs below this portion of the brain, with only 80% nerve function, are not going to do as great as they otherwise would. And over time, when cells in the body produce over and over again, eventually a problem arises.

One lady had breathing problems for years and couldn't inhale without an oxygen tank. After her very first adjustment, she took her first deep breath in years!

You need help, so who do you go to? Let's say you go to a medical doctor. They usually don't know what's going on so they wind up getting blood tests, which indicate something's wrong. Well no kidding, you know something is wrong, that's why you're there in the first place!

The only people that are specifically trained to detect and fix this small injury and look for these small interferences are chiropractors!

Now, the interesting thing about the body is that, every second of our life, the body produces 2.5 million cells. I know, an incredible amount isn't it?

So if you have a particular area of the body where the nerve is not functioning at a 100%, you might get 2.5 million cells as usual—but this time, they wouldn't all be normal!

You might actually get abnormal cells in that particular area of the body. And that's a real concern, because let's say the nerves around the head aren't working efficiently, over time, a patient might develop headaches. They also could have sinus problems. All as a result of this missing 20%!

I am not supposed to say this, however I will anyway to prove a point, why is it that many of my patients have the same problem in their spine with the same condition? I practice this specific scientific method of spinal correction called the Pierce Results System and we use video X-ray.

There was a time when I was real confident in my abilities to help people and correlate their spine to their disease. One time I took five patients and told them I was going to look at their spine and tell them what they have. Then I would do their history and ask them what their problem was. I was 90% accurate. This scared me in seeing how accurate their problems were related to their spine.

Medical doctors would, of course, look at the head or the sinuses in order to correct the problem. Yet the problem has started elsewhere, so how can that cure anything? Imagine stepping on a dog's tail. The dog would bark but the dog is not having a vocal cord problem, it is a tail with a foot-stepping problem. If you remove the foot off the tail the dog stops barking.

That's the reason why a lot of people simply don't have much luck when it comes to the medical community; they are given drugs to help offset the pain, but aren't actually cured underneath.

So, of course, the problem keeps coming back and back and back

I am not God. I do not have magical healing powers; no doctor worth their salt would ever claim that—and if they do, make sure you carry right on walking! Interesting to note that if you put all the best doctors in the world in one room, they together couldn't create one living cell! But I do believe that our knowledge of chiropractic can be used hand-in-hand with God's inner healing to give us the very best chance at health.

The power of a specific Chiropractic adjustment catapults our own inbuilt natural healing; in a society that often gets carried away with new technological developments, it reminds us that the laws of nature are still the most important rules to live by in order to stay healthy and happy. Humans are the only animal that takes pride in the development of its society, but throws out years of knowledge at the same time.

It may surprise you to know that of the hundreds of patients' testimonials we have, only a very small percentage is related to back and neck pain. We see when problems of the lower spine create menstrual cramps get removed these patients with cramps got better.

That's because chiropractic has an impact on the entire body; what we do to correct your spine can help organ problems, allergies, cancer, heart disease, and high blood pressure, among other things—things that are generally thought of as incurable. Yes, in some cases, we see illnesses that patients have had to live with for the past 10 or 20 years simply disappear!

Want to know how we did that? Keep reading.

But first, before we go any further, let's take a look at how chiropractic got started in the first place because it's a pretty amazing story in its own right; it is also the best introduction to this unknown and misunderstood science that I can give you because it illustrates the far reaching benefits of the discipline perfectly.

Let's take a close look at exactly what happened on September 18 1895, the day that changed the world and chiropractic was born...

THE AMAZING HISTORY OF CHIROPRACTIC

On September 18, 1895, a magnetic healer called DD Palmer was working in a small town called Davenport in Iowa, when his first client was a man called Harvey Lillard. Lillard had been hard of hearing for 18 years. A rich man, he had been to the best doctors in the world only to be told, time and time again, that there was no cure; he would remain deaf until the day that he died.

On examination, Palmer saw a big lump on Lillard's back, a bone that looked out of place. Curious, he asked if he could put it back in.

Why did Lillard say yes? Perhaps because he had exhausted every other option and thought things couldn't get any worse.

Palmer had no idea what he was doing but simply popped the bone back in; it seemed like common sense. And do you know what? It worked!

Three days later the patient returned with 100% restored hearing. Amazing!

Ironically, Palmer thought they'd found a cure for hearing loss! He advertised it and a people came from far and around for this amazing treatment, but Palmer soon realized that sometimes the treatment worked and sometimes it didn't. In some cases, however, while the hearing issue remained, other ailments were cured - even heart problems!

That's when Palmer started to see the potential in his discovery and when research into chiropractic first started. It was the first time in history that a man used the spine as a lever. And the discipline to heal the entire spine with a specific force. Only before that time manipulation was used to aid the body, but without a rhyme or reason.

Now, let's take a pause here and take a step back. Some readers may wonder if I've just made up this incredible story, or if I've exaggerated it for a special effect. (I didn't and I'm not, by the way!). How can clicking a bone back into place cure hearing loss, I'm sure you're asking. Is it even possible?

Well yes, it is. Why? Because everything is interconnected!

The way we help people is that we do something called a specific *chiropractic adjustment*.

An *adjustment* is actually a method where we get these bones, off struggling nerves which are slightly out of place, back into place. What a lot of people don't know is that there is a difference between *manipulation* and *adjustment*.

WHAT IS MANIPULATION?

Imagine playing pool or billiards; if you take the white ball and hit the rest with force, one of them might happen to go in. That's a manipulation. You just put a force in the body and tons of things move into place but not necessarily the right ones.

WHAT IS AN ADJUSTMENT?

This is very specific, very precise and for a particular reason. It's like working out the angles at pool, and hitting just one ball with the white ball in order to put it in the corner pocket. You know just how to hit it and where, and with how much force, to achieve the result that you want.

Believe it or not, most physical therapy or osteopaths manipulate joints in this way and do not adjust. They do what's known as a manipulation where they grab the neck and twist it to the right and left, just hoping something falls into the right place.

It's a little like a dentist pulling out all the teeth in the hope of finding the one with the cavity! Whereas an adjustment has more finesse; you are going after one particular problem that requires handling and fixing and correcting it without causing any problems for the rest.

Note: In choosing a chiropractor be sure to choose one that adjusts, not manipulates. There is a definable difference between them, your health is on the line.

Chapter 4

Why it's Not Just About a Pain in the Neck

A lot of people mistakenly think chiropractic is only about curing back or neck problems.

That's because chiropractors advertise it that way in your local phonebook and they do not understand how interconnected our entire body is; they do not appreciate just how much our nerve system keeps us healthy—or not, or how a simple bone out of place in the neck can actually cause a physical reaction elsewhere in the body.

Of course, a chiropractic adjustment will certainly be beneficial for back and neck problems, but my experience has taught me that it has much more far reaching consequences.

I have seen it help people with migraine headaches, carpal tunnel syndrome, shoulder pain, as well as problems with organ function, and even Crohn's Disease, which is a very debilitating disease of intestines.

It can also help people with heart problems and high blood pressure.

As a matter of fact, that's why I got into chiropractic in the first place, because of my father's high blood pressure. Let me take a moment to tell you his story because it really changed my life forever.

My Dad's Story

My father had had high blood pressure for as long as I could remember; at the time he was in a very stressful job and situation—which hasn't changed much—but he was taking up to 10 medications a day for high blood pressure. And the medication's, its side effects. This was something he would have to check religiously throughout the day with his blood pressure cuff and his black notebook.

I was a personal trainer at the time and I was very confused; my belief was that you fix everything through exercise and diet, to eat more supplements and vitamins. Yet dad took the medicine route, which I respected, but it simply wasn't working for him.

I had just started working with this chiropractor and so I said: 'Dad, you know, chiropractic might be the thing for you! I thought chiropractic was about back pain, but in this chiropractor's office I saw testimonials of real people that got better. One had high blood pressure.

He didn't believe me, of course. He was as skeptical about chiropractic as I was, but after weeks of me hounding him, telling him to Go, Go, Go, he finally agreed to get a spinal chiropractic examination which luckily took x-rays to see inside the body. I actually told him up to 20 times. He said chiropractors weren't real doctors and that the spine is not the problem. He had no back pain. All of the common considerations that occur before seeking that first chiropractic visit. I saw real testimonials that should help my dad's ailing condition. A condition that he, his excellent medications and "I got the best medical doctor" couldn't fix!

The truth to him was that medicine, his idea of a real science and his little opinion of chiropractic which wouldn't work was the end of the discussion. Regardless, his opinion left him sick. If the truth shall set you free then well he was soon to be DEAD wrong! Dead from those drugs and weak heart. In the simplistic right or wrong logic something had to be wrong. Was it his opinion and medicine or was it chiropractic and proven testimonials?

So after these 20 times of asking he finally gave in and I finally got his exam. My dad then came back for his report of this exam. This doctor found a problem on his x-rays. The doctor showed a normal healthy x-ray where the bones were aligned and compared it to my dad's x-ray. It was off! My dad saw a shifting in his spine. He thought how could this be? I don't feel a problem! The person I trust the most to my health, my medical doctor, never told me there was a problem! Then the next x-ray was put up and there it was again another problem! Undeniable evidence something wasn't perfect in my dad's health. He figured there was nothing left to do but get this fixed. My dad then got his first chiropractic adjustment. So my father started getting adjusted by this chiropractor, and a couple of months went by.

As I said, my father would take up to 10 medications for this high blood pressure but one day, he started to notice that he felt a bit weird; he noticed this Blood pressure was going down, just to be careful, he went back to his medical doctor—the one who put him on the medication in the first place—and the doctor said: 'This doesn't seem right! Maybe these medications are too much!'

So he switched him from 10 medications over to 8.

Now, at this point, I'm thinking: This is amazing! My dad's life is starting to change—he's got the same job, the same diet—but his body was changing!

This is what got me interested in chiropractic. I applied to chiropractic school after doing my undergraduate degree and got accepted.

I started going and becoming a chiropractor, and was seeing the same results that this chiropractor was showing on my father.

Now, this chiropractor was using one of the old traditional ways of adjusting the spine. It was working well, but it was when I finally got my father over to this other doctor who does this method called Pierce, and the results were truly amazing. It was almost a miracle!

My father went from taking 10 medications a day, to eight, then six, and then four!

It eventually got to a point where he was worried—maybe because he was checking his blood pressure throughout the day—that his blood pressure was now TOO low!

So he went back to his medical doctor, the one that put him on these medications, and he carried out some typical stress tests.

He did all the stress tests and so forth and they put him on the EKG. My father came back for his results a few days later and what he said to my father actually changed my life. A real shocker!

The first words he said to my father were: 'What happened to you? Did you walk through the fountain of youth?'

He said: 'I've been a cardiologist for 25 years, and I've never seen anything like this!'

So my father obviously explained that he was using chiropractic and his son is in chiropractic school etc.. etc.. This doctor was amazed. He said: 'I've never seen something like this!'

So, to cut a long story short, my father finally gets off all of his medication about six months after this examination—ironically, around that same time, this medical doctor, who was taking the same medication, actually had a heart attack and had to leave practice!

I was so happy that my father no longer had to take his medication; not just because of the freedom he now had to enjoy his life, but because of the side effects.

As part of chiropractic school, we can actually get more education than the medical doctors in anatomy and so forth. But there are also classes that we can take to learn about medications.

Obviously, with my family interest, I wanted to know exactly what it was that my father had been taking—and now I had the ability to research it.

I got a list of all his medications he had about 20 of them over the years, and I did my research; that's when I learned that side effects aren't really side effects at all—they're actually new diseases. I printed out a stack of papers, literally about a half-inch thick of his medications and their side effects.

So I wrote him a letter; it was the most powerful letter I have ever written to anyone. I put it in the mail with this write-up, and I sent it to him. And he gets this letter, and this is how the letter read.

I said: "Dad, if it weren't for chiropractic, instead of you reading this letter, I'd be reciting it over your grave."

I knew the next step of hypertension/high blood pressure, a heart attack and death.

Chiropractic saved my dad's life and right now, my dad is over 67 and he actually bikes over 10 miles on his bike!

He hasn't had to change anything in his life either—he has the same job, he eats the same foods and does the same exercises; the only thing that changed his life was a specific chiropractic adjustment.

That's the thing that really keeps me passionate—because there are people like my father out there that don't know that these medications can cause them problems, or that there are natural, safe options instead that could actually help them PERIOD! It's not about an opinion its about hard-nosed facts!

I firmly believe my father's life has been saved as a result of chiropractic; he is one of my proudest patients. He's been under my care now for nine years and been off his medication for 14.

He tells everyone this story and, as a result, a lot of people that he's told, or who have heard about him, come in and end up getting the same or similar results that he did!

For me, that's an important part of chiropractic; teaching people how they can improve their health both while they are in my office and when they're at home.

Our goal is not just getting people out of pain but to make them healthier.

That's why I have written this book; to demonstrate that getting back to nature—avoiding medicines where possible, and trying to live stress-free lives—can make a huge difference to our health.

Living by the principles of a non-invasive treatment like chiropractic can also help ensure that our bodies can continue to take advantage of the God-given healing that makes us so very special. God didn't give us any extra organs so we have to look after the ones we have.

I'll also go into how nature can help us cure allergies, colds and even help with weight loss and childbirth.

Before I move on though, let me tell you about a interesting study into chiropractic and hypertension that has had amazing results. The study looked at the results of chiropractic adjustments on people with early stage high blood pressure. The results were so astonishing that chiropractic featured in the *Journal of Hypertension* for the very first time, highlighted as a more successful form of treatment than all the other hypertension medicines and treatments. It would be nice to see before those drug commercials "before trying this drug with its side-effects try safe non-side effect chiropractic." *Maybe in my Dreams!*

Study 2—Journal Of Hypertension

HOW: Of the 50 people in the study, half were given a very specific adjustment of the Atlas vertebra, the bone at the very top of the spine, while the rest were given fake sham adjustments. The patients were unaware of which group they belonged to.

WHAT: Eight weeks after undergoing the procedure, the 25 patients with real adjustments had significantly lower blood pressure than the 25 'sham' patients. Their blood pressure dropped by an average 14 mm Hg in systolic blood pressure (the top number in a blood pressure count), and an average 8 mm Hg drop in diastolic blood pressure (the bottom blood pressure number).

The research also noted that there were no side effects of chiropractic adjustments.

Testimonials

"Since I received chiropractic care, I have felt less pain in my neck. I have gotten more sleep than I used to get years ago. I have felt less light headed than I used to as well, and I have been able to think more clearly than I used to as well."

D. H.

"Prior to chiropractic adjustments I would get a lot of neck pain as well as headaches. Currently I am under chiropractic care which has helped with neck pain as well as headaches. The wellness talk educated me in regards to the spine and the way the human body reacts if injured."

A. L.

"I have a nagging shoulder injury from playing ice hickey. I have been under care for several years, but recently I came to the office with shooting pains from my shoulder to my fingers. I was holding my arm because I could not let it rest in its natural position without pain. Dr. Spages adjusted me and the next day I was pain free and had complete motion. Now I can play ice hockey again against Dr. Spages wishes."

M. L.

"My name is Gloria and I have been treating with other chiropractors for about 5 yrs. Just recently I was sick and lost my voice. The next day I was seen by Dr. Spages and he adjusted me, I can tell you that, that same night I felt better. I was able to sleep and I woke up feeling better and my voice was back. Now my cold is gone and I feel more relaxed. Dr. Spages did something that other chiropractors had never done before and that is making me feel better and seeing an improvement. I am thankful that I have met Dr. Spages."

G.T.

"After years of excessive drainage in my left ear following mastoid surgery, the drainage has become less. In response to my question to my ear specialist as to why he thought this was finally happening he simply

said… "I guess your body has finally decided to heal itself" I immediately thought to myself… "I'm sure this is due to good chiropractic care."

L. G.

"In the month of August my menses were horrible. Excruciating cramps, bloating, headache was so unbearable I called out from work. My appointment for Dr. Spages was that day. I was gonna cancel the appointment because I was feeling so bad. I kept my appointment. Dr. Spages knew I wasn't feeling well. I told him about my bad cramps. He gave me an adjustment and told me he could press on a nerve that will relieve the pain, but I would be mad at him because it can hurt. I told him to do it. Afterwards, the next day I felt better. The month of September menses was so much easier. Hardly no pain at all. Thanks Dr. Spages"

T. T.

"Every winter I suffer from several colds with major sinus pressure. These usually last several days to weeks. This year I only had one cold that lasted more than a day, and it was gone the day after my visit with Dr. Spages. The pressure in my head was gone in about two minutes after my adjustment. I should have seen Dr. Spages sooner. This is the healthiest winter for me in over ten years, thanks to Dr. Spages."

J. A.

Chapter 5

Why it's Not All Cracking and Popping:

What Is the Pierce Results System?

Some people have a fear of chiropractors because they think they will start cracking and popping the bones in the neck and cause more problems than they cure. They might have a point.

It's been found that some chiropractors do not adjust but do what we call spinal manipulation—moving all the bones in the spine around in the hope that the one problem bone will slot back into place in the middle of it.

It's the billiard ball analogy we talked about in the last chapter—hit the balls with enough force and one may well go into the pocket.

It is best to use more finesse—both with your billiard games AND chiropractic care!

I use a version of chiropractic called the Pierce Results System. This uses the more careful spinal adjustments—looking at bone by bone by bone—that I mentioned previously.

Remember: the better billiard player assesses the angles, has a plan and chooses which ball to hit where. Once he has his target, he carefully works out where to hit the ball, how hard and with how much force to roll it slowly into the pre-picked pocket.

The Pierce Results System is actually practiced by only about 20 certified doctors in the entire world, 18 of those in the US. In the area that I practice, New Jersey, there is only one other practitioner.

The key benefit of the Pierce Results System is an important one to our patients; they enjoy the fact that it only takes a handful of adjustments to correct the spine.

In some cases, I can do in one visit what it would take other chiropractors 15 to 20 visits to do. **The Pierce Results System is all about getting immediate results**. Sick people are sick of being sick.

Don't get me wrong; I firmly believe in using chiropractic as you would a dentist. Common sense tells us that you should visit your dentist every six months for regular check-ups in order to keep your teeth in good order; wait until you have tooth ache and there is already a problem. However, visit your dentist before you have problems and hopefully you'll avoid the need for any invasive treatment at all. I remember I saw a movie where someone asked "When did Noah build the ark?"… "Before the storm!"

That's what I propose to my patients; come to see us and have chiropractic adjustments regularly, and we can ensure that your spine never develops any problems.

What I do believe, however, is that patients with *existing* problems shouldn't have to wait for 10, 20, 30 or even more adjustments before they start to feel better, or before the adjustments have a positive effect. Ideally they will start to feel better immediately.

So we try to focus on the areas of spine which have the most problems and fix those. This style doesn't do any twisting, popping or bending; remember, that's the equivalent of smashing the pool balls and hoping for the best.

Instead we do a straight adjustment which directly goes right towards the bone and gets the bone right back in place as quickly as possible. We look to actually put a misaligned bone back into a normal position. It's a very effective method.

When we're looking for one misaligned bone we're looking for all different things such as up or down, right or left, on a right angle or left angle, and believe me it is not as easy as it sounds.

The Pierce system applies very special rules that must be obeyed to ensure results.

My Own Story

You might be curious how I first became aware of the Pierce Results System of chiropractic. I have trained in the Pierce Results System of chiropractic for over 13 years. I also held the office of President of the Pierce Results System club for 2 years.

They say that doctors make the worst patients and that was certainly true of me; like a lot of my patients, I suffered from a problem in the spine throughout early adulthood—namely, a subluxation, a misaligned bone that puts pressure on the nerves and reduces the body's ability to heal itself correctly.

I found that this could be a very dangerous thing. After going through a lot of research on this, I knew I had to find the most scientific means of getting this fixed.

I used several different chiropractors, and what did I learn? I learned that some methods could supposedly adjust and correct my spine, only to be told by another practitioner that there was still a problem.

At school I had the opportunity to see very different methods right after each other. I felt that if this was serious, then there should be one application that fixes it. Eventually, after searching more than eight different methods of chiropractic, I came across Pierce Results System, which is the method I currently use.

The amazing thing was that, after studying and researching this method for a long time, I finally went to my first seminar and I met Dr. Pierce Jr. the son of Dr Pierce; he was introducing this method to a wider audience. He showed us X-rays after x-ray of unfixable problem patients FIXED, and we could see people getting better overnight. Yes really, OVERNIGHT and even some in a few minutes!

I was just blown away by the changes that I saw in people's X-rays; problems that, with other chiropractic methods would not fix.

It just really fascinated me. So finally I got my first adjustment done by Dr. Pierce!

The following week, I went to another seminar on all these other different techniques, still learning and researching and I found that I was the only person there that didn't have a problem with their back!

Each room there was filled with over 60 chiropractors, as well as chiropractic students and patients—and I was the only one out of all these that didn't need care!

It was just incredible to me; it was the most powerful demonstration that I've ever seen. It also made sense to me, much more than traditional chiropractic if I'm honest.

In chiropractic school they taught me to compare one bone to the next bone. It sounds ok in theory, but I had a problem understanding the effectiveness of this method because it's possible that both the bones were affected and needed treatment.

What if we are comparing one bad bone with another bad bone? That surely can't be right, but unless we look at the entire spine, how can we tell?

Whereas with the Pierce Results System, we look at getting a bad bone back to its normal state—where it's normal state is defined as how God created us. That's surely foolproof and much more effective.

Learning about all of this and seeing the results, I said to myself: 'You know what—they really have something to this method!' and that's when I really went into it.

I learned it from Dr. Pierce's son (also known as Dr. Pierce), and then I eventually taught advanced methods at Life University—the largest chiropractic school in the States—and that was truly a great experience. I actually had teachers that were teaching me during the day, while I was teaching them at nighttime in this advanced method—and it was really rewarding.

When they saw the difference—what Pierce can do in one adjustment compared to traditional chiropractic, which often needed up to 30-60 adjustments to attain the same results—they were really elated.

For me, Pierce is the answer because I don't think it is fair that patients are constantly given the wrong information and are told to take drugs that aren't necessary. They're told that there is no help.

When a patient goes in a hospital in extreme pain obvious pain and at the hospital they spend 2,000,000 dollars of the best research, 500 years of connected practice and at the very end they say " there is nothing wrong" Are you kidding me?

I'm sick of this. I am totally fed up and I'm taking action to go out there and teach more doctors about this method so that the patients can get better and people don't have to resort to using drugs and medication without getting any real help! You need a system to get well and that should be the only intention not insurance.

A doctor's intention is to always get a patient well or at least it should be—even those doctors who over prescribe drugs or misdiagnose still want to help people but imagine if you had a tool, a powerful tool that does it better than the medical drug and surgery system that would make a big difference. Better health naturally with our own god-given healing ability.

So, let's get down to the nitty-gritty here.

What really makes Pierce Results System different? How do those billiard ball analogies really work in practice? What do we do in the office that you wouldn't experience in a chiropractor of a different discipline?

Chapter 6

Why All Doctors Are Not the Same:

The A-B-C of Pierce Results System

The first thing we do when you walk through the door (after saying hello, of course!) is to find out what your problem is.

When you're looking for the cause of a problem, you want to get down to the core of what is making the person sick. We spend a lot of time finding the problem; until we know this, how can we best treat you right?

By understanding what your problem is and where it comes from, we can make sure our treatment is targeted and specific. All of which means much quicker results for you and a blessed relief from any pain!

It's like an investigation. It's almost like you are putting on a detective hat to go in there and see what's wrong with the person. So you need to know a few things before you begin.

The first one is 'where is the problem?' At first, the patient tells us which organ has the problem so we already have an idea. Then we look for the nerves which connect to that area.

So, if a person tells me he has a heart problem, I will look for the nerves that control the heart. In chiropractic, we look for the cause of a problem while, as I've mentioned before and will keep mentioning time and again, medicine looks at the effect of that problem on the body. It's a classic case of the tail wagging the dog, so to speak.

We look at the nerve because the nerves control every cell, tissue and organ of the body. It's amazing how every single cell of the body is touched by a nerve; it's as if the nerve is a puppet master and it controls the body.

When the body isn't functioning correctly—usually because of stress—that's when problems arise; we see them first in the spine and then we very often see them later in the organs.

So the first thing we look at is 'where' the problem is.

A lot of times that's funny, because sometimes patients come in and ask: 'Do you want all the reports from all my other doctors?' And I say to them in a funny way: 'Yeah, that'd be really great, but how many doctors did you go through, with that information that you didn't get better from?'

And they would sit there and say: 'Three or four'. Sometimes they quote as many as eight.

So I say to them: 'Let's use the latest technology to actually find if there's a problem that could be helped through chiropractic care in this office'.

So, how can we find out your problem area with such certainty? How can we tell you much more about your body than you even know yourself?

We can do this by using the most scientific methods available...

We Take a Video of the Inside of your Body

We use special instruments such as video fluoroscopy; an instrument that is very uncommon in chiropractic, but exceptionally useful. Video fluoroscopy is actually a motion picture of the spine. You really get to see a video presentation of what's going on inside the body. Many chiropractors don't use this instrument because a) you need special training to use this, and b) the equipment is quite expensive.

We Take a Blue Print of your Spine—*look under the radar*

We also take a blue print of your nervous system EVERY single time we see you! This is a special kind of instrument—*thermography*—that shows us if your body is healing. This is particularly important if you have had adjustments in the past because we want to see if it is working. Part of the reason for this is so that we know if your problem area needs further treatment, or if we should stay away from it. Chiropractors have been traditionally know to over adjust. This tool is my policeman to make sure I follow the pierce notes.

That's the bigger question isn't it? When do you stay away from a condition? Not necessarily when do you go *in* there, but when should you stay *away*? *Is* the body healing?

When a person breaks his arm, he would take an eternity to heal if you tapped his arm every single day and asked him how he is doing. So Joe how are you doing? Smack, so Joe how's things today? Snap! So sometimes, the best plan of action is to leave it well enough alone so that your body's own internal healing—which we kick started for you in the last adjustment—can do the job that it is supposed to.

I think that is an important point to mention as well. Good chiropractors, ones who really know their stuff, won't tell you that you need an adjustment if you don't.

Of course, not all chiropractors have the advantages of the techniques and technology that Pierce uses in order to ascertain that, but those that do can learn if your body will benefit from treatment.

We're driven by the desire to help, not to make money!

So we do a very thorough examination and you'll be surprised how many times things are missed just because people don't have the right technology, or are not looking in the right place.

HOW THE PIERCE RESULTS SYSTEM CAN CHANGE LIVES

I had one patient who wasn't able to cry, as her eyes did not produce any teardrops. If she needed to look to her side, she had to turn her head.

Her eyes were dry and painful and she was very self-conscious; something so simple impacted on her life in many different ways.

Within three months of getting adjusted, she was doing a presentation on her grandchild and suddenly she was in tears. She hadn't experienced that in years.

Can you imagine how powerful that was? No one has ever welcomed tears with as quite as much enthusiasm.

This was a woman who had lived with this condition for many years and was made to think there was no remedy for it.

And do you know why that was, why she had all but given up hope of ever living a normal life? Because every single doctor she had visited was a medical doctor and no one thought about fixing her spine!

All those years wasted, in pain and searching for a cure, when all it really took was three months of spinal adjustments to change her life for the better.

So, let's look at the techniques and instruments used in Pierce in a little more detail:

- **Our Crystal Ball**:

  I've already mentioned our technological equivalent of a crystal ball. In this system we have a graph called *thermography* that determines how the body is healing. Even though all chiropractors try to ensure that there is no pressure on any of the nerves in the body, Pierce does it slightly differently.

  We use this instrument to learn which areas of the body are not functioning at a 100%. If a person is getting a chiropractic adjustment, we want to make sure that body heals before we go and do something else to it.

  This is very interesting because we can see inside the body without surgery. So, this is the first tool that tells you when and where to adjust. It's very powerful.

  Even medical doctors always don't know when to prescribe medications and when not to. With the help of this instrument we're able to know whether there is any area of the body that is receiving too much stress and should be left alone.

  As a doctor, you want to help heal but you could also do *too* much; there's just no way of knowing.

  Let's say you take medication every day. You are supposed to take 5 milligrams of this particular medicine at 8'o clock. What if at that point of time your body doesn't need that dosage of medication? What if it needed only 3 milligrams instead of 5 milligrams? How can you know that? Answer: You can't.

  You just have to go on taking the medicine without knowing whether your body needs it or not. In this way, you can make your body go crazy. So this tool is very important for letting us know whether or not a person needs chiropractic adjustment or not.

- **Motion X-ray of the Spine**:

  Next up, we have the amazing motion X-ray of the spine that I've already touched on, the *video fluoroscopy*. It's the most advanced way of finding if there is something actually wrong with the spine and uses low radiation to see if the bones are moving correctly.

  Think of it as looking at the engine of your car running without having to open the hood.

  You can actually see how to body is moving inside and how it is functioning.

  Compared to traditional X-rays, it's extremely safe, thorough and detailed. It's a tool that I feel I couldn't practice without. If I took a picture of someone, you would just see them for one second, that's what a regular x-ray does. It is just for a second, and it would be hard to figure out what happened. Say for example, you see a picture of Larry Bird taking a jump shot. So the question is what just happened. Did he just let the ball pass, did he steal the ball, is he practicing, is he playing during a finals game. You don't have a lot of the story. But if I showed you a thirty second clip of Larry Bird shooting the basket ball, you have an exact idea of what happens. And that really defines the difference between a regular x-ray and a motion x-ray. In a regular x-ray, you get only one second, but in a motion x-ray, you get many seconds, you get so much more of the story as opposed to that just one little second.

- **Regular X-Ray:**

  Like a lot of medical doctors, we do use regular X-rays, but it's how we analyze them that makes the difference. We compare these X-rays to a normal human being—what a perfect person should look like. It's almost like having a spinal engineer. The art of chiropractic is the utilization of chiropractic as a natural path to true health. I could pick up a knife; it is a tool to cut fruit, vegetables etc. But that same knife to a skilled chef could create a prize winning meal.

- **Palpate:**

The next in the order is a tool we use our own senses, this is not as reliable but it's a tool that can tell us what's wrong and can put a finger on the exact problem. I became good at palpating when I did drill of putting a hair underneath yellow page sheets. As I turn more and more sheets over this hair I gained a better tactile ability. Much like a blind man hearing, or a deaf girl seeing! Despite the very good skill I attained I still don't use this as a great means of finding the problem. Being human I could err which my tools won't.

- **No hands!**

We have something called 'instrument adjusting' which enables us to heal areas where hands cannot go. It's like a fine tuning instrument that we use to help patients get back on course.

- **The Pierce Analysis:**

Our instruments ensure we have the best technology at our disposal but that would be of only limited benefit if we didn't know how to use it.

The Pierce Analysis ensures that we have the best minds at our disposal; this more than anything helps to make sure we don't miss anything.

Dr Pierce had a great idea; he got some of the greatest chiropractors of his time—all of whom had done what he considered to be the most effective adjustments to patients—and created one system out of each of their ideas.

So every time we look at a patient we have a combined knowledge of the greatest minds in chiropractic. What an all star team!

It's the best of the best!

So, Who *Was* Dr Pierce?

Let me tell you some more about Dr Pierce himself.

Dr. Pierce was one of those people that were always searching for answers. Back in the 70's, he was looking at doing what is known as *upper cervical* adjustments.

This adjustment uses the top bone of the spine—the *Atlas*—as a lever. Hence it is called the *Atlas adjustment*.

Pierce noticed that a number of his patients were not getting better; there is nothing worse as a practitioner than not being able to help people.

Finally, he met another gentleman who was doing research on another bone in the neck called the C5 bone.

As Pierce looked into it more, he noticed that the C5 bone dictates the other bones in the spine by controlling the spine and helping it maneuver. That was a breakthrough discovery.

After a lot of research, he was successful in adjusting this bone in a way no other doctor ever had. He adjusted it from the back as opposed to twisting the neck as most other chiropractors would do. He had more changes to show on X-ray, than any other doctor available.

Dr. Pierce won the chiropractic contests held at Logan Chiropractic College every year. He got the worst cases of *scoliosis* (spinal curvature) fixed with the least number of adjustments.

We're talking about before and after X-rays here that are mind blowing. It's like putting a wrecked car into a car wash and the other end being back to normal.

The ability to correct severe problems without surgery is a gift of Pierce chiropractic. In this analogy, it's like going as far as *changing* the oil of a car without opening the hood!

Our three step approach to Chiropractic Helping Patients

Let's treat ourselves to the time to summarize exactly what we've learnt here about the Pierce Results System of chiropractic.

It's no secret that there are three crucial steps to chiropractic helping patients, so what are they?

- The first thing is the 'know how'. Using all our knowledge, along with X-rays etc..., before you do anything to the patient; plus, taking an 'after' look after an adjustment to see the change— that's number one.

- The second would be the ability to actually use the tools to take advantage of this 'knowhow'—it's very important.

- The third step is actually being committed to doing number one and two! Having the endurance and the passion to do this is really important.

Just as the doctor of Pierce Results System looks at the entire spine to ensure everything is in order, so I like to look at the entire body. You'll see that in later chapters as we come to talk about allergies, weight loss, colds and much more.

I constantly strive to educate my patients about how to stay healthy. There is so much bad information out there, so many healthy ways of living that we have rejected because of technology and new developments; people should get the truth. They understand why their body is not healthy so that they can make the right decisions.

Only then, can they truly enjoy the good health that you deserve!

Testimonial

'I thank God for the Pierce Results System'

Rev. Pollard and his wife Barbara both enjoyed Pierce chiropractic

My Wife's Story

Rev Pollard: *I first heard about Dr Spages' practice after an interview on the radio. A friend of mine, who knew that my wife Barbara had been gravely ill for the past three years, gave us a tape of a program they had heard on WFME radio. I took it home and put it on my desk.*

It stayed there for a couple of weeks until I got a call from the same friend asking about what I thought of the tape. So, finally I listened to the tape and while listening to it I began to praise God.

Tears began to fall because I felt that here was the answer that we had been looking for.

My wife had been totally confined to the bed with 24 hour care for the past three years and had been sick for more than six years.

We went to at least 10 hospitals in the area and they couldn't tell me the reason behind her illness. All the major hospitals and doctors in this metropolitan area could not tell us what was happening and why she was having excruciating muscle spasms and why her nerves were dying out.

Chiropractic is not as painful as a lot of people believe it to be.

It gets a bad reputation, but it's certainly worth trying.

It could change your life!

One hospital had said that Barbara was a 'good case'. I had no idea what this meant, but really it meant they had no answers. After they conducted all the tests, they said everything was okay with her.

Another hospital suggested that it was all in her mind and there was nothing wrong with her body. They said she can walk if she wants to—she just won't do it!

Needless to say, we disagreed with this prognosis.

Barbara wanted nothing more than to walk, but she simply wasn't able to. She was unable to move her feet and arms and we were assigned to pain management doctors since the doctors couldn't tell us what the real problem was.

After I heard about Dr Spages, I convinced my wife to go for a visit; after all, at this point we had very little to lose.

We got an appointment and Dr. Spages took us through the regular intake system and carried out a motion picture of the spine. Looking at the condition of my wife's spine he said "I don't know if we can help but we'll try."

He said he thought my wife would benefit from a spinal adjustment, so we thought we'd try it. I had high hopes, of course I did—my wife has been living in pain for six years—but I was also a little wary. We had been promised hope before, but with very little results.

What I will say, however, is that from the very first adjustment, my wife began to feel relief. It was amazing.

She had been wearing a collar for about six years that the doctors had given to her in order to keep her headaches down. After her first adjustment, she didn't need the collar anymore as the headaches had gone! It really was that quick.

She also had what is called a frozen shoulder. The doctors had put her arms in a sling to keep her shoulder from moving and her shoulder froze. Her neck bones went out of place because of the brace.

She started chiropractic adjustment a little while ago, and I'm thrilled to say that my wife hasn't taken any pain medicine for the past five months!

I'm giving God the glory for Dr. Spages and Pierce chiropractic. I am the biggest convert and its biggest fan.

It has been my desire to get as many people involved as possible in the Pierce Results System because I truly believe it is life changing. Dr Spages came to our church and presented the program to our congregation. As a result, we already have about 25 people from the church enrolled in the program and others are still coming.

Now let me just say something about those people. This number includes people who couldn't move without their walking stick before they went to Dr. Spages; now they're coming up the church stairs without walking assistance! I have never seen such big smiles.

My wife was the greatest testimony for the people in our congregation. When they saw Barbara being able to lift both her hands—something she couldn't do for years—that was enough to make a lot of them enroll in the program.

We just give God all the glory for the changes this form of chiropractic has brought about in our lives.

My wife no longer needs to be totally lifted from the bed. She can move out of the bed herself with the help of a transfer board. Earlier, she couldn't lift her arms and couldn't do anything.

Now she is cleaning the house, packing my bags when I have to travel and everything else that she used to do before she fell ill.

We're still trusting God that one day she'll get off the wheel chair and walk. That's not so important.

The most important thing to us was 'What is causing the condition?' No one could tell us. So when Dr. Spages showed us on film what was causing the problem, we were satisfied that at least we knew the cause.

Would you believe that before this I didn't even believe in chiropractic?!

That's why it took me two weeks to listen to the tape. At that time, we were making preparations to go down to John Hopkins Hospital in Maryland to see if they could help Barbara. If they couldn't, we'd have gone next to Duke University in North Carolina.

We weren't going to give up, but I shudder to think what Barbara's life would be like now if we had done that instead of going to see Dr Spages.

My Story

Rev Pollard:

At the same time as my wife signed up with Dr Spages, I signed up for myself as well. I had high blood pressure—it had been 264 over 112 at one point in time—but I still didn't think there was anything really wrong with me.

Little did I know! When I looked at the X-rays, I realized that my spine was just as bad as my wife's!

Each time you go in to Dr. Spages' office, they get a graph done. Before he does anything, he examines the graph to see what's going on in your system and because of that, he knows exactly what has to be adjusted.

He wouldn't stop adjusting and checking the graph until it got to the point where he wanted it to be.

Finally, when I asked him what he saw, he told me that I had pressure build up on my brain and he couldn't allow me to leave his office with that.

He saved my life by discovering in one visit that there was pressure building up on my brain.

I've had adjustments since and now I'm running a normal pressure of 120 over 60 or 70—that's down from 264. I still have to take pills periodically and monitor my pressure, but it is much better now.

One day I took a tablet when I shouldn't have; I'd just got adjusted—that and the pill drove my pressure down too low!

It truly is amazing what chiropractic can do. Not only did it help my high blood pressure, but it helped in other areas too.

I had developed phlebitis in my leg. After my first adjustment I went home and discovered that I could lift my leg and put it into the pants once again.

It's strange how such a little thing can really make your day seem brighter.

Chapter 7

Why Did I get sick?

With Everything We Already Know, Why Do Regular Doctors Ignore the Spine?

I've already talked a great deal about this amazing thing called our spine and the nerves underneath it; it truly is worthy of respect. Along with the brain, it is responsible for the health of your entire body.

And you thought it just gave you aches and pains every so often!

If you didn't catch it earlier, the father of modern medicine Hippocrates told us to look at the spine as a pre-requisite for dealing with any illness. He knew more

Sickness is a process. No one gets fat overnight by eating the wrong food; obesity takes time.

The same goes for sickness. People are given the wrong information about their health.

than many of our current doctors! He said look to the spine it is the requisite for many diseases, which is written profoundly in my office.

Now, I want to talk more specifically about *exactly* what can happen to our bodies when even one part of the spine is out of alignment.

When I first started learning about chiropractic, I was astonished by just how much we already knew about the spine and the nerves beneath it; even as far as to be able to say that this one particular bone *here* will cause a problem *there* if it is out of alignment.

Of course, no spinal adjustment is ever the same on two different people; what can help with hearing loss in one person, for instance, can do something entirely different in another. We've seen that already in the history of chiropractic, haven't we? And yet, we can still pinpoint to incredible accuracy which bone is responsible for sinus problems, for instance, or which bone is out of alignment and causing kidney problems.

If someone comes to us with a specific health complaint, we know exactly where to look first—that's because we know which areas of the spine correlate to, or link to, which areas of the body.

It gives us an extraordinary power to be able to correct all sorts of ailments and diseases in the human body.

So, let's take it step by step and bone by bone...

Slowly moving down the spine

Think of...

WHERE YOUR HAIR MEETS THE TOP OF YOUR NECK

If there is a problem in this area, patients can show up with headaches, or sometimes they have difficulty sleeping. The top of their neck is also related to sinuses; this is the area where people get their sinus problems from. Think also dizziness, head colds, allergies, runny nose, vision and hearing problems.

They catch more colds when there is pressure in this area.

PRESSURE AT THE CENTER OF YOUR NECK

If there is pressure on the centre of the neck, people suffer from a condition called *carpal tunnel syndrome*. This area is also responsible for a stiff neck, tennis elbow, lung and breathing problems, as well as asthma and chest pains.

Additionally, this area controls the thyroid gland. So, people sometimes go on different diets and different things to improve their body physique but if that gland is not working correctly, they have a really hard time.

WHERE THE COLLAR SITS ON A SHIRT

Moving a little further down the spine, we see that this is a vital area because it's here where the nerves go to vital organs—namely the heart, lungs, breast tissue and chest. This is grand central station.

Any problems here can affect areas connected to breathing, or blood pressure. Common problems include high blood pressure, bronchitis, pneumonia and congestion. Sometimes we see patients with high blood pressure or kids with asthma. When we notice that women have breast cancer or lumps in the breasts, we always look at this area in order to find the cause of the problem.

THE NERVES IN THE CENTER OF THE BACK

By the bra strap

When there's pressure on the nerves in the centre of the back, it affects the gall bladder or causes reflux or causes heart burn. It can also cause liver problems, gallbladder, stomach troubles, heartburn, diabetes, acne, pimples, and gas pains.

THE LOWER PORTION OF THE BACK

It would seem obvious that the nerves in the lower portion of the back should go down to the legs, as well as making their way to the reproductive organs and the intestines. When we see patients suffering from ailments such as constipation or sciatica, knee problems or ankle problems, we know we must look to the lower part of the spine to see if everything is functioning correctly. The lower part of the spine is also responsible for hernias, low back pain as well as poor circulation in the legs, sciatica, constipation, chronic tiredness, diarrhea, infertility and menstrual cramps. Chiropractic always works. Always! If you are not getting results don't blame chiropractic blame the chiropractor.

If you still doubt the power of the spine, consider the example of Christopher Reeves (Superman). This great man broke his neck while horse riding. And what happened?

- **He couldn't move his legs**; he hadn't actually broken his legs but because he had broken his neck, he wasn't able to move his legs.

- **He needed a machine to help him breathe**. Again, didn't break his lungs.

- **He had another machine that helped his heart function**. It's the same result here too; he didn't break his heart, he broke his neck.

So, one major fracture at the top of his spine made his whole body shut down.

Picture it like a stream with a dam; water—or in Christopher Reeve's case—information, simply couldn't get past this obstruction.

So because his lungs weren't getting the order to breathe, or his legs to walk, or his heart to function on its own, they were incapable of doing so.

Forget the Bark; Get off the Dog's Tail

It is so simple when you look at the Christopher Reeve example isn't it; it's so easy to see what must be happening to the body inside, but people still don't fully grasp it. Even medical professionals continue to ignore the spine.

Believe it or not, Hippocrates, the father of medicine, said back in 360 B.C that you should look at the spine; it is the cause of many diseases.

But what do we see? Now, close to 2000 years later, most doctors still don't look for the actual cause of disease in the spine—they look elsewhere. It's like, if you step on a dog's tail and it barks (which of course, it will do!) a lot of times people go and look exactly at the bark—they look at the vocal chords of the dog, and so forth to try and see what is happening—but truthfully, you should be looking at the tail.

In actual fact, what you *should* be doing is getting your foot *off* the poor pooch's tail RIGHT NOW! Until you do that, the pain is still going to be there and the dog will still continue to bark.

Once you remove your size nines from the poor dog's tail, the dog stops barking.

A lot of times people don't look for what's causing the pain— for example, we talked about carpal tunnel syndrome earlier; when there's pain around the wrist, people look immediately at the wrist.

And that, in that analogy, that would be the dog barking—but a lot of times, where the tail is being stepped on, the real problem is in the neck area—that's where the whole thing stems from, in terms of the nerves and so forth. And a lot of people don't look for that.

Even if medicine doesn't appreciate the importance of the brain and spinal cord, nature certainly does. After all, they are the only organs that are actually encased in 'stone'. This protective 'stone' is, of course, your skull and your vertebrae.

I'll give you another analogy: sometimes, I ask some of the women at my presentations—if you had a million dollars, where would you put it? The smarter woman would say, obviously, in diamonds, gold and so forth, but realistically, they put it in a secure bank. And that's exactly what the body does—it puts the most precious organs in our body, which are the brain and spinal cord, inside of a secure bank called the skull, and the spine.

I've already explained how the brain controls everything we need to actually function. That signal goes from the brain through the spinal cord and the nerves, which passes those signals onto other parts of the body, telling them what to do. Again, we've seen this with the Christopher Reeve example above.

Chiropractors look for little areas in the spine where there is any kind of blockage. Just to reiterate, we're trying to get information from the brain all the way down the spine and if there is even one percent of stoppage on the way, you can understand that the rest of the body won't be at a hundred percent. It'll only be at a 99%. Overtime, that's going to show as a symptom.

Let's look at health from total health to death from a distance.

- Health
- Stress

- Subluxation

- No symptom

- Symptoms

- Suffering

- Death

Of course sometimes these blockages don't show as a symptom and that's the really scary part; if you see no symptoms, how can you fight it? Some of the leading causes of death in America have no symptoms. Look at heart disease—in better than 50% of the cases, the first symptom of heart disease is sudden death! Another symptomless illness is cancer. One minute you're feeling great and the next thing you know you have a lump in your chest and you have two months to live. And there's no symptoms there!

This is something that never fails to surprise me, no matter how many times I hear about it. When you do something as minor as stubbing your toe, you feel instant agony, right? As a child, your first experience of it is so severe and unexpected that it almost feels like you were going to die, doesn't it? And yet, we don't even feel something like fatal cancer which can destroy you. That's so weird isn't it?

DON'T BE A PAIN IN THE NECK

Let me give you a typical example of how chiropractors think, particularly chiropractors like myself that use the Pierce method. Say you came in to see me with a lower back pain problem. You might be surprised when I tell you that this probably actually started in the neck. Yes, that's right—as contrary as it sounds, your lower back pain is probably a result of a problem in your neck. And when you understand how, it will make complete sense.

Lower back pain often starts with a whiplash injury, falling, and car accidents; then over the years, the spine slowly starts changing—the neck becomes what's known as 'straight neck' or 'military neck.' From there, the mid back becomes straight, and then the lower back eventually loses its curvature.

Let's say a person, for easy numbers, weighed 100 lbs—well, they should easily have all the weight equally shared in every one of their bones and their spine. However, when their spine straightens out as demonstrated above, the pressure becomes uneven and they get too much pressure in particular areas; it is these areas that cause problems.

Now most people can relate to a bulging or herniated disc. Believe it or not, it's really from a bone out of place. And it often starts way before the original occurrence happens. So if they bend over to pick up a pencil from the ground and feel a pain in their back, they think the <u>pencil</u> did it. Of course, a pencil has little to no weight to it, and really the problem was a result of the spine degenerating, and not being fixed at an early age.

That's why we have children from two days of age getting adjusted—because, you know, sometimes the birth process is very traumatic. Not to mention that as the baby grows up, he or she is passed around with everybody holding him, as well as him/ her trying to hold his or her own head up with these tiny little muscles. If we don't help them now, they will be suffering in the future!

Needless to say, the only way you can fight back against these symptomless illnesses is to make sure your spine is in the best shape that it possibly can be, to ensure that there is nothing out of alignment, no bone pressing on a nerve that could cause a problem for you one day. We look out for you *before* you feel a symptom.

Benjamin Franklin—"An ounce of prevention is worth a pound of cure."

The above example demonstrates the difference between medical doctors and chiropractors; can you imagine going to your medical doctor about a pain in your lower back only for him to start looking at your neck? Not likely to happen is it? He's more likely to either look at the lower back or give you some pain killers to ease the agony.

Medical doctors and chiropractors get similar schooling before they branch out into their respective disciplines, so medical doctors are not taught to think like we are. If a person comes to them with pain, they are looking for the pain and not the *cause* of the pain.

Let's face it, if they found out what caused the problem, they would be losing money too wouldn't they? Medicine is a multibillion dollar industry; those behind it don't want chiropractors to take away their livelihoods.

The medical community would come to a standstill if the doctors started concentrating on the cause of a problem and not the symptom. Because maybe, just maybe, they would cure it and that patient would never have need for drugs or medical intervention ever again! Where's the money in that? It's like teaching someone to cut their own hair.

I personally believe that is one of the reasons why I see a lot of patients who come to me as a last resort. It's actually a running joke in the office, but patients often go through as many as eight doctors before they actually come to us, and it's not that the other doctors weren't doing a good job—it's just that they were looking somewhere different for the source of the problem.

These patients have done what they think they should; they started off with traditional medicine, but despite the doctors' visits and the drugs and the examinations, they just aren't getting any better. They might have drugs to help them alleviate the symptoms but those drugs can cause even more problems than they started out with.

Go ahead and ask an asthma sufferer if they would rather not have asthma, or if they're happy to live with their inhaler? I bet I can tell you what they would say!

Earlier in the book, we talked a little about hypertension and how chiropractic adjustment can help ease the problem. As we're examining specific illnesses in this chapter, it only seems right that we talk about it again in more detail.

One thing we see all the time in a person with hypertension is a subluxation in the spine.

The World Health Organization defines a chiropractic vertebral subluxation as: "A lesion or dysfunction in a joint or motion segment in which alignment, movement integrity and/or physiological function are altered, although contact between joint surfaces remains intact. It is essentially a functional entity, which may influence biomechanical and neural integrity."

That's a lot of long words, which essentially all add up to mean that there's a problem area in the spine; a blockage which prevents full functionality of the areas beneath.

The bone in question here is called the *Atlas, the very first vertebra in the spine.* In Greek mythology, Charles Atlas used to hold up the globe; this *Atlas* is a little three ounce bone that holds up a 10—12 pound head!

Yes, it's a little bone with a very big mission.

Adjusting this bone takes special training, special analysis and viewpoint, because it's one of the most important bones in the body. That bone has kind of a manual of its own on how to take care of it. There is upwards of 16 methods to adjust this one bone. It's that important.

This bone plays a huge role in the body because it controls the respiratory and the heart rate centre of the brain.

So if this bone is under pressure, it can affect the heart rate and that's where high blood pressure comes up. The other thing is kidney function; there isn't much medication available to help kidney function.

Most of the people who suffer from high blood pressure take some sort of *beta blocker*. *Beta blockers* are like mini heart attacks; they force the heart to do something that it doesn't want to do.

Many times when the kidney blocks up, there is pressure behind the kidney function. If the kidney is clogging, the blood has to go somewhere.

As my father can testify, if you start taking pills for high blood pressure you will notice that after a few months you're on nine others, taking your total to 10 pills—and you're no healthier than you were before you went on medication. So you are actually walking on a very thin sheet of ice.

That's why specific chiropractic and spinal adjustments can help those who suffer from hypertension, and a whole host of other diseases. Life can truly be enjoyed when you're at your healthiest and happiest!

Testimonials

After visiting Dr. Spages for two months I no longer suffer with cramps. Before I came here I was doubled over with pain from my monthly cramps and had to take painkillers for at least three days.

As of now I have not even taken as much as an aspirin.

I feel great, have not been sick and have a lot more energy.

M.K.

I suffered from severe seasonal allergies, for which I had to take all kinds of medications; these in turn caused all sort of side effects.

I also suffered from headaches due to sinus pressure.

My biggest problem was the horrible backaches that I would wake up with everyday.

I had tried just about everything to deal with the pain, but it would only treat it for the moment. With the first three adjustments, my allergies went away, along with my headaches, and I felt so relieved!

My backaches have diminished significantly and I feel healthier with more energy.

I thank Dr. Spages for this, not only because his method is great, but also for his love and true devotion to chiropractic, which makes the real difference in the healing process!

D.M.

I came here feeling pain in my shoulder and no strength in my arm.

Since chiropractic I feel much improvement, especially after leaving the office after my adjustment.

I recommend that anyone who feels pain should seek adjustment ASAP to avoid prolonged pain and lead a free life.

F.G.

Chapter 8

Happy Times = Sick Times

The one thing that chiropractic teaches us is to look at the whole body when it comes to our health. Our entire body is interconnected in ways that are amazing; imagine all the orders that your body needs to follow in order to work every day. Move this, move that, regulate this, regulate that, push this here, remove that from there... your body is the most incredible engine on earth.

Remember what organ first develops in a fetus?

If you said the brain, well done!

Ok, so next test: think of all the organs necessary for survival within the body. Now have a guess at what part of the body develops immediately after the brain? Is it the heart, the lungs, the kidneys? They're crucial aren't they? Well yes, they are. BUT more important still is the spinal cord.

All of those orders are coming from your brain. The way those orders reach the areas they need to, is via the brain's 'tail'—your spinal cord. The spinal cord passes messages from the brain to your peripheral nerve system and beyond. Chiropractic recognizes just how important that spinal cord is to your health and wellbeing. Nature does too; that's why it is protected. The brain and spinal cord are so precious and valuable that they are the only part of the body encased in 'stone'—you know it as the skull and the spine.

The principles behind chiropractic show us that through adjustments and pressure removed from the spinal cord, we can correct problems all over our bodies. When any bone in the spine is under pressure and stress, it gets misaligned. A misaligned bone can bring the body's efficiency down from 100% to as little as 40%. There's no way that won't affect your health. Perhaps one or more of the nerves within that cord has an impact on the organ they connect to, and hey presto! You have a health problem.

It really is that important. The good news is that by working with the spine and making those *adjustments* we talked about earlier, it can bring you back to good health and ensure you stay there. And isn't good health the cornerstone of everything that follows? Keep healthy and you open yourself up to love, family, success, happiness… all the great things that life has to offer. All are possible if you have good health. You can certainly enjoy them a lot more anyway!

From our understanding of the principles of chiropractic (there are 33 principles!), we now know more than ever before about how the body works and how to keep it healthy - and these are tips I'm going to share with you right now.

Have you ever finished work for a longed for vacation only to come down with a cold? Or looked forward to the holidays only to end up feeling a little under the weather? Annoying isn't it?

It doesn't have to be inevitable, however; once you appreciate why you're always coming down with a cold, or feeling run down at certain times of the year, you can fight back.

Let's take one of the most stressful times of the year—the holidays.

A lot of health issues show up around the holidays. Why? Because there's a lot that your body has to cope with during that time, including climate change. One moment you are outside in the cold and the next you're inside the house where it's hot. It's not actually the cold weather that causes the problem per se; it's that your body has to adapt to changes in temperature several times a day. That's a lot of work, and a lot of stress.

Yes, there's that S word again. S-T-R-E-S-S. Remember what I told you in chapter one; all doctors, no matter their branch of healthcare, agree that stress (lack of 'ease' in the body, 'dis-ease', aka disease) is what makes people sick.

Add to that, the fact that people tend to stop exercising around the holidays AND over-indulge in food they shouldn't be eating—not to mention the stress of finding that must-have doll your daughter wants this year or spending money you don't have—and you can see where I'm going with this. Stress, stress and more stress.

Your body is a great machine, but it needs some help from you; it can tackle stress IF you're eating well, exercising and looking after yourself, but if you're not...

Let's look at the three ugly faces of stress:

Physical Stress

This is the amount of stress our body has to physically deal with; it can be a result of something basic like incorrect sitting posture or sleeping for eight hours on a bad mattress or as a result of a major fall or a car accident, or anything similar. Our bodies are hardy things but they do get bashed around a lot, even in everyday life. Add the holidays to the picture—physical stress due to the weather changing, the risk of slipping on ice—and it all builds up. Sit in the wrong position for any period of time and you'll start to feel it more and more. Imagine it like the snowflake effect; putting one snowflake on a branch doesn't weigh much but snowflake after snowflake after snowflake after…you get the picture, and eventually it'll bring the whole branch down.

Even things you wouldn't expect can cause physical stress to our bodies. Women's high heels, for instance, can cause back problems from misalignment; even the weight of some of your purses are incredible. I have a special scale to illustrate how heavy it would be. My record 12 lbs! As well as causing a bad spine, these things also reduce the benefit of correcting a bad spine if you're not going to give them up.

Think also of someone who sits in front of a computer screen all day; people who do this tend to slouch. The slouching affects mostly the base of the neck and the lower back. Pressure at the base of the neck affects the heart and blood pressure and pressure in the lower back affects the kidneys which are the filter of the body. It also affects blood pressure. All this just because you work in front of a computer! All of this affects your body via physical stress.

All humans except for the few NASA astronauts have gravity as a never ending stress.

By the time a person reaches 30, think about how many car accidents, sports injuries, falls, bad mattresses and pillows etc can affect the spine.

Chemical Stress

We're living in a chemical society nowadays; there are more chemicals around us and in our food than ever before. Artificial flavoring, preservatives, colors, pesticides, antibiotics… you name it and they add stress to the body. Your body has to work to address each and every one of these. It's a tiring job.

Emotional Stress

Some would argue this is the biggest stress of all; generations of men and women told they can have it all has resulted in a huge amount of pressure being heaped on us. Anything can cause emotional stress and it doesn't just have to be the obvious work-related problems. Especially around the holidays, travel, traffic, shopping, dealing with relatives or even coping with the weather alone can all cause a considerable amount of emotional stress.

How can the body handle all this stress? That's where chiropractic comes in; handling excessive stress that happens to the body for any of the reasons above—or the 101 other potential reasons we face every day. Think of a chiropractor adjustment as a stress zapper.

Of course, there's a limit to what any doctor can do without the patient taking responsibility for their own health. As a doctor I can give you advice but I won't be there, day in and day out, to make sure you take it. Your doctor can recommend the ways to get proper nutrition but he can't actually be there to cook your food for you. .

There are five key tips for good health, and only one of them is the doctor's responsibility. The rest is yours. What are they?

Top Five Tips for Health

- **Proper Sleep**—your body recharges itself when you sleep. Some people will need the full eight hours, some will need less; some will even need more. The rule here is if you don't wake up feeling good, you probably need more sleep. Try to go four or five days without sleep and you'll see how important it is; they torture prisoners with sleep deprivation! Sleep recharges your battery.

- **Proper Nutrition**- We're going to talk about this a lot more in the Weight Loss chapter but let's just say that there's a big difference between diet and nutrition. Diet is anything that you eat so if you eat peanut butter and cigarettes than you have a peanut butter and cigarette diet! This is why there are so many books based on someone's opinion of what you should eat. But nutrition is something you put in your mouth that your body actually *uses*—the vitamins and minerals it is able to absorb. There's a whole range of reasons why humans suffer from digestive problems, all of which we'll come onto in good time, but for now let's just think about it. Isn't it true that the only animal which cooks its food is human beings? Are we also the only ones that have problems digesting our food? Yes, to both counts. Your body craves vitamins and minerals and if you're not giving it what it needs, you are going to stay constantly hungry.

- **Mental Capacity**—We've already mentioned emotional stress; whatever goes through your mind goes into your body. A negative person is doing their body harm as a direct result of their negative thinking. You program yourself depending on what you put in; if you put bad stuff into your mind, you get bad stuff out into the body. A child, for instance, will have a hard time resolving a conflict if all he sees and learns is violence on TV and in music.

- **Proper Exercise**—This is the big one. We all *know* that we should exercise, but for some reason we're not doing it. Something seems to get in the way. We can do anything today as long as we have a bathroom and an internet connection; we can make money, order food, pay the bills, talk to one another without leaving the house, and much more besides. That's why kids today sit for hours and hours in front of their computers and never see the outdoors. We have kids who are obese at 13. Our own society is making us unhealthy.

- **Proper Nerve flow** - This is the *one* responsibility of the doctors, particularly chiropractors. Your nerves control *everything* in your body—every single cell, tissue and organism in your body. It's a mind-blowing idea; your nerves controlling your body instead of the other way around.

So let's say you're trying to *lose* weight but a bone is putting pressure on your thyroid gland; it's never going to *happen,* or at least not to its full potential. Or you're trying to sleep but your nerves aren't sending the right messages or telling your body to create the right hormones; it's going to be impossible to get good sleep. Conditions such as depression are caused by a misbalance of dopamine in the brain; this is your nervous system not performing as well as it should.

If your nervous system isn't working great then there is no way you're going to have a good mental attitude. One bone out of place in your spine can put pressure on a nerve going to the legs; in turn, you may lose some of the strength in those legs. A second could be the difference between gold or nothing. You may get an injury as a result. Everything - and I do mean everything - stems from your spine; that is why chiropractic is so important.

But don't just take my word for it. Ronald Pero, from New York medical research department, found that cancer patients have an immune system that's 200% weaker than people without cancer. This is true. In contrast, people who have been under chiropractic maintenance care for five years have an immune system that's 200% stronger than those who are not under chiropractic care. That makes them 400% stronger than cancer patients. That's a staggering statistic. Imagine if they put that on CNN or Fox News; there would be lines for miles outside chiropractors' offices.

I see it all the time. We've seen that patients' immune systems get stronger incrementally each year. If we're talking about colds, as we are in this chapter, we'll see a patient with say 15 colds in their first year. The next year it's usually half that, the year after that half again and so on until it's virtually nil. It really is a miracle.

THOUGHT FOR THE DAY:

THE BEST HEALER INSIDE ALL OF US IS GOD.

We already produce the things we need to heal a great deal of injuries; if we twist our ankle, for instance, it swells; this acts as a cast to prevent the area from getting worse. Stress interferes with that amazing process. Stress causes bones to misalign, which in turn puts pressure on the very nerves they are protecting. That's the cause of bad health

---

Testimonials

*I began visiting Dr. Spages after visiting another well-known doctor for **Tennis Elbow**. That doctor wanted to give me medications for my pain, which didn't help the pain at all. I went to Dr. Spages and he was able to reduce the pain after only four visits. I have no pain now and my tennis elbow is feeling much better with no medication. I recommend anyone see a chiropractor before considering a traditional doctor. Chiropractic has relieved pain in my back that had been there for almost 20 years.*

As a football player I've encountered numerous injuries just on my shoulder alone. I was about to get surgery on my shoulder but Dr. Spages had informed me that just by adjustments alone I wouldn't need the surgery. I gave it a shot and within weeks I felt looser and less tense and most important of all I didn't really have any pain. I am doing activities I wouldn't be doing if I had surgery.

M.J.

Chapter 9

Tackling Allergies Without Drugs

Getting people well is easier when they can simply lay down on my chiropractic table and get adjusted. However, when a person has allergies they may be sneezing and experience some difficulty breathing which could make it harder to adjust them. Allergies can make a person's life miserable.

Whether it be hay fever, an allergy to dust mites, pets, food, or something entirely different, it's something you have to live with EVERY SINGLE DAY. What's more it's still not appreciated by the general public at large for the sheer agony that it can be; non-sufferers, for instance, tend to think of people with hay fever as sneezing every so often and that's that.

They don't see them when they wake up in the morning with their eyes almost welded together because they're so swollen; or have to watch them as their eyes stream all day. Sneezing too is not just an inconvenience; it can be a physical pain as pressure builds up in the sinuses.

And let's not forget that a great many of these allergies can also trigger life-threatening asthma—and a lot more besides. Nowadays we're seeing more and more diseases and illnesses occurring as a result of a weakened immune system—and what causes that weakened immune system? You got it! Allergies!

It's a big problem in this country; allergies are the 5th leading chronic disease in the U.S. among all ages, and the 3rd most common among children under 18. The annual cost of allergies is estimated to be nearly $7 billion. That's a heck of a lot of money. But what are allergies, really? Why do some people suffer and not others? What do allergies actually do to your body, and how can you tackle it?

Simply put, an allergy is something that a body can't handle. To be more specific, the brain and the nervous system can't handle it. Allergies are considered to be foreign to the body so it tries to attack them. It's not, as you might think, a case of your body being underactive, but the exact opposite—your body is going to war, trying to attack something that it doesn't understand.

I see many patients with allergies that are at the end of their line; they've tried every other form of healthcare or help and it just hasn't worked. And that's not surprising. For most disciplines tend to only look at the end result; they look to stop the sneezing or the breathing problems. They don't take the time to look at what is actually causing the issue, what has gone wrong in the body, in the first place. And if you don't address the core reason for the allergy, how can that person ever really be truly healthy?

For many people, their allergy means having to pop pills every day, because that's what they have been conditioned to think they must do. People are brainwashed into believing that they need medications for every problem. By the time we're 18 years old, we have watched more than 18,000 hours worth of drug commercials. That's brain pollution on a huge scale!

The problem with taking medications is that medicines do not actually increase your ability to become healthier; medicines are chemicals at the end of the day. That's why a great many people are also allergic to the side effects of medication. People always take medication in order to tackle allergies, but that's not the correct answer! Just because you are seeing a drug commercial that doesn't mean that it's right. One needs to get to the root of the problem to see what's causing the allergies. Our experience has been that people are sick of taking medications for allergies as they make you feel awful and there are worse side effects associated with it. So, they try to handle the problem anyway they can.

First, they try to avoid whatever is causing the allergy. That may give them relief for a short while, but really, they're not taking care of the real cause behind the allergy - they're just avoiding the allergens. Should someone be allergic to air? Yes there are more pollutants but if it was strictly absolutely positively the pollutants every single person breathing that air should and would be sick. It's as drastic as a hay fever sufferer never going outside in the summer so they don't have to deal with the pollen. Their body isn't getting any better, but their life has just got a whole lot worse! As a result, the body continues to weaken.

Then they start taking over the counter medications. This goes on for 3-5 years or longer and only serves to further weaken the immune system; it isn't long before it starts to damage other functions of the body as well, such as the different organs. From there, they go to medical doctors such as Ear, Nose and Throat specialists. The doctors try different things like clearing up the nasal passage and this goes on for some time.

At this point, imagine how you'd feel if this were you? Maybe it *is* you. So let me guess; you probably feel exhausted right about now; you've tried and discarded every single thing the medical community tells you can help you and it hasn't worked. How can something as simple as an allergy cause this much discomfort? All you know is that you can't let it continue; you have to find relief somehow, and that's when you maybe start to think of chiropractic.

True Story:

There was a time when I had a pretty decent spine. I was actually under Pierce Chiropractic care. In fact, in school, we always got free care from other students, but I always paid for my care, knowing how valuable it was. So, I used to travel pretty far and go see a doctor who was doing Pierce Chiropractor in Georgia. My spine was looking really good. It took me some time, but I finally got it to the point where it was looking great, and I actually had some nice curves in my spine.

I got into a pretty bad car accident. I was driving down the road and a car got in front of me, and I couldn't stop. He was actually cutting over an intersection. It was the guy's fault, but I hit the guy as I was going forty miles per hour. I remember this happened on a Friday. I went to the hospital, they checked my x-ray and ironically they were surprised at how nice my x-ray was. They were actually shocked at the curve in my spine. But the fact that there was a curve in my spine after the accident was even more of a shock. So that was pretty interesting!

Now, over that weekend, I happened to go outside. I went in an area where there were a lot of woods. I found that I was constantly sneezing over and over and over again. And I never had such a sneezing bout. And I was never allergic to anything! After this accident, there was a point in time, with no exaggeration, where I sneezed nearly 30 or 40 times in a row.

My face was completely red and my whole face was numb as a result of sneezing so much. I did that all day.

On Sunday, I stayed inside, not wanting to see anything that was going on outside. And finally on Monday, I actually changed my classes around, so I could go get adjusted. And I got adjusted on Monday. And I got 90% better after that adjustment from a Pierce doctor. By Thursday of that week, I never had allergies again.

So, it was so weird that in a matter of less than a week, between a Friday to a Thursday, I went from having severe, severe allergies, and couldn't handle any pollen to before that never having it and after that never having it. It really shows how there is a relation to symptoms and people's sicknesses right over to the spine.

Picture the moment when that person finally comes to a chiropractor and we find out that there's actually a problem in their spine—which no one ever looked at before. Imagine their blessed relief if we can cure their lifelong allergies with an adjustment to their right bone in the right direction at the right time and like a miracle—healed.

The simple fact is that most people don't know what chiropractic is, so let me tell you. Chiropractic looks at getting the body better from within; it works towards allowing the body to heal correctly without any unneeded intervention. We don't look to remove any organs or add any chemicals to the body.

All types of chiropractic work with the inner healing of the body, which is known as natural intelligence or the "inborn intelligence" of the body. The body is an incredible thing; it always knows exactly what it needs to be healthy. The question is what causes a person to fall sick in spite of that? The answer is stress—and as you'll hear time and time again in this book, that's the one thing all doctors can agree on!

Chiropractic looks to correct the consequences of that stress so the body can do the healing it is meant to do without intervention. It is what we call an altered science—you never get the same result twice. Medicine is also not an exact science. Person gets a drug, and gets better symptom next person gets the same drug and gets worse and next person takes same drugs has reaction and is hospitalized. That is not so exact. I could adjust someone on a particular bone of his spine—let's say his neck bone and I could see the problems in his big toe getting fixed. On another person, the same adjustment may take care of his allergies. There are tests we can do to identify the underlying cause of a great many illnesses, but before we come onto that, let's take a quick look at the common causes of allergies right now.

What Causes Allergies Today?

There are a lot of factors that contribute to allergies today. They include:

- **Pollution:**

   There are more pollutants in our air than ever before. How can there not be, when there are more cars on our streets and a lot more factories churning out God knows what? An estimated 50 million Americans suffer from all types of allergies—that's one in five Americans. The real question is whether the amount of pollution we have accumulated over time can ever be undone. To my mind, that's a very tall order.

- **How We Look after Ourselves**

   People simply don't take as much care of their bodies as they used to; that's a fact. They may not even know it but if you look at the diet of an average American, it's full of artificial flavors, additives, sugar, and flour—their diet is predominantly processed foods. This weakens the immune system. Nowadays, an allergic response isn't just restricted to a sneeze or a rash either; it's getting much more serious than that. People are getting other symptoms such as diabetes type II, migraine headaches, rheumatoid arthritis, colitis which is inflammation of the intestines - all possible caused by allergic responses and food sensitivity. You might have seen heart palpitations, seizures, ulcers, mood swings, hyper activity, joint swelling and appetite changes—all these things happen as result of allergies.

Chapter 10

Fix the Person Not the Air

When a patient comes to us, we need to know certain things—it's like an investigation. It's almost like you are putting on a detective hat to go in there and see what's wrong with the person. You need to know a few things. First, you need to figure out where the problem is. Traditional medicine does allergy testing or blood work to tell us 'what is wrong' and that something is wrong. This testing doesn't know <u>why</u> "what is wrong" is there in the first place.

If the person tells us a certain organ has the problem, we know where to look first; we look for the nerves that connect that area. So, if a person tells me he has a heart problem, I will look for the nerves that control the heart. We look for the nerve because the nerves control every cell, tissue and organ and system of the body.

Every single cell of the body is touched by a nerve as if the nerve is a puppet master and it controls the body. It's incredible! When the body has stress and isn't functioning correctly, that's when problems arise; they start first in the spine and then go out to all these organs via the nerves. So the first thing we look is 'where'.

We also use technology and tests (the ones I mentioned in the chapter on, "Why All Doctors Are Not The Same") to look at how a particular part of the body is healing, and the *rate* at which it is healing. Remember I told you that the body's natural instinct is to heal itself; we need to see if that is happening and if not, why not?

Hippocrates, the father of medicine, used to put clay on people's body. The areas that dried up the quickest were the areas of concern. If it was around the heart—heart problems, around the lungs—lung problem and so on.. he knew how important the spine was. All that time ago!

We stepped this up in the pierce results system with NASA technology of infrared heat which gives us a reproducible print out of what areas of the body aren't healing. If you can identify the parts of the nerves that control allergic reaction, you can also keep a close eye on how well the problem is solving itself. Once you remove the stress factor, of course!

How Can You Identify the Source of *Your* Allergy?

As well as identifying the cause of the allergic reaction within a body, it's also useful to identify the particular allergen that triggers it. That's not always as easy as it sounds. If you're having an allergic reaction to food, for instance, you may not know which type of food is the culprit. That's because you may not get an allergic reaction right away, depending on how severe the allergic reaction is.

People with severe allergies—anaphylactic shock, for instance—tend to know what it is that triggers the problem as the reaction is almost instantaneous, but in many other cases, the reaction can happen slowly and over time.

True Story:

Some years back, I brought my office manager to a seminar with me in Florida. Some other staff joined us later. The night we got there my office manager and I went to dinner at a seafood restaurant. I didn't know this at the time, but this office manager had been allergic to seafood, especially shellfish, her whole life. She had been hospitalized before and had to take special shots for it, or she could become deathly ill.

She didn't order any seafood, but still warned me that she had to watch out, and that she had her emergency pen back at the hotel just in case. I on the other hand did order seafood, but made sure none of it touched hers.

We started to eat. She was very cautious the whole time, even though she only ordered chicken. After a few minutes she noticed her face beginning to itch, and couple of seconds later, her face started to swell also. She told me that she was not feeling well, and that she may be having an allergic reaction. We realized at this point that her chicken must have touched seafood at some point during its preparation. She decided to try to hang on a few more minutes, but, as time went by, her throat started to close. Now we were scared! We were halfway through dinner, but I called for the check immediately. I just wanted to get her to the room so that she could get her medication. I didn't know how to handle it; I had never been in this situation. It's not like I ever had people eating seafood in my reception area. It wasn't something that people usually go to a chiropractor for.

As we were walking back to our hotel, which was only a few blocks away, she recommended that I give her an adjustment. I told her we shouldn't waste any time, and that we should get her back to her room to get her medication. She insisted I do a quick adjustment for her.

I had seen my fair share of miracles with chiropractic, and even though I was worried about getting her back to her room I agreed to adjust her since I knew her misalignments. I couldn't adjust her the way I would have liked to, being that the only platform I had to work with was a nearby park bench. I adjusted her neck, and then we continued toward the hotel right away. I was walking very fast, but she began to walk slowly behind me. Then suddenly she stopped me. I said, "no, we have to keep going, we have to get you your shot." She said, "No Dr. Spages wait, my nose stopped running, my face is feeling better." I didn't believe it. I kept walking.

By the time we got back to the hotel all symptoms of the reaction were gone. I was in complete shock. I expected her to get really sick; she was 33 at the time and had this allergy her whole life. One adjustment made that big of a difference. She never took her medication that night.

Before that incident I never thought that the spine would have an effect on something like food poisoning. Chiropractic never seizes to amaze me. You can have a chiropractor walk into an area and help people with just their hands.

As a patient who is not currently visiting a chiropractor, you can do your own allergy test. If you are exposed to something that you are allergic to, you don't have to wait for the obvious physical symptoms; you can instead measure your heart rate. Your heart rate will increase as a result of having some sort of allergy, even before you see the external results of it.

Now, typically, what happens is that if you eat a food that you suspect may be causing some sort of allergic response, you have to wait maybe 15, 30 and 60 minutes. In each of those times you actually check your pulse for one minute. This is called your base pulse. It's sort of like the Boy Scout test—eat the food—wait—if you get sick or die it wasn't good for you! If this starts to rise, you are having some sort of an allergic response. That's one of the tests that people do in order to know whether their bodies are going through an allergic response. You can do allergy testing through blood testing such as the IGG test which is a very good blood test. It is a little expensive but I know it to be the most accurate.

You also have to look at what kind of allergies you're getting. Runny nose, coughing, headaches, fatigue, sinus congestion, sore throat, skin rashes - all these things could happen if you are exposed to allergens and sensitivities. Pollen, mold, food, animals or even regular air pollution can result in allergies.

In chiropractic, we're actually looking for the causes of bad immune response. People say they feel better after having adjustments to their spine; there are over a thousand cases where people have come in with some sort of sniffles and after we've adjusted them they were already feeling better.

The immune system and the nervous system work hand in hand. As a result, it can take some time to get the immune responses back; the immune organs are slow response organs. We see people getting a lot better over time.

When we see a patient who has been under care for at least two years, their allergy symptoms fall off remarkably as their immune system gets stronger. As I've already mentioned, however, we don't just look at today's symptoms. We look at the nervous system to see if you have allergies and we check that the nervous system is working correctly. Let's say that you got rid of your allergies but your nerves aren't working correctly. Eventually, this will give rise to another problem, perhaps even another allergy. So, you may be killing a dwarf but you have a giant behind it! Medicine stops here; chiropractic helps you to slay the giant so you need never have allergies *ever* again! Well done sir sniff a lot.

Testimonials

I came here with Sciatica and the doctor helped my pain and suffering since May 1, 2003. I chose him over an orthopedic doctor because I didn't want injections or surgery. I tried this and liked it. He's very comforting and worthy of going to see no matter what the cost. I express this to my whole family and friends frequently. I suffered with lower back and neck pain for months.

Only after a few visits with doctor Spages did my neck and back pain stop. I started to notice that I have more energy and I sleep a lot better. Dr. Spages' care and passion has encouraged me to strive harder to eat more nutritionally, exercise more and have my spine adjusted on a regular basis. I feel great.

M.K.

It didn't hurt as much as when I go to the gym! My biggest amazement was in the springtime. I usually experience severe allergies that I couldn't take anymore. I noticed this year that my allergies were not as strong as they have been in previous years. Years before I had asthma, I was sneezing a lot and my eyes would become itchy and I would develop a runny nose; now most of these symptoms are almost gone, thanks to the adjustment I received.

C.B.

Chapter 11

Fighting the Flab:

The Real Reason You Can't Lose Weight

Besides the spine there are other factors to health. A big problem is body composition. It is harder to be aligned when their center of gravity has changed. Weight loss: It's the big, fat elephant in the room. We might talk about it but, as a nation, we sure don't seem to have found the answer to it. Nearly everyone I know—male and female—has been on a diet at some point in their lives, often more than one, but we just seem to keep gaining those pounds.

I know it makes more than one person in this great nation of ours miserable. And who wants to spend their lives being miserable?

A lot of people simply don't understand what they are putting into their mouths, or why. Even those trying to eat healthily are still piling on the pounds, and that's surely not fair, right? So, why is this happening?

Simply put, it's happening because we have forgotten our history, the way our bodies have always worked; nowadays we are subjecting them to more and more technological advances that might improve our convenience and way of life, but do nothing for our bodies.

There's a lot that nature has taught us about our bodies and how they work. Let's look at what our bodies are doing when we're gaining weight.

Sometimes the body simply doesn't function well enough. What do I mean? Well, the first thing we need to look at is the difference between nutrition and diet.

Diet *is literally what you put in your mouth.*

So, if you eat pencils and cigarettes, you're on a pencil and cigarette diet!

Nutrition, *on the other hand, is about putting things in your body that it can actually use. I'll repeat that again; nutrition is what our bodies can actually* use. *Our body craves nutrients such as vitamins and minerals—we need them to grow, to be healthy, for energy and life—but all our technology has only made it harder for our bodies to absorb these nutrients.*

Humans are the only animal that cooks its food; it's no coincidence that we are also the only ones to have digestive problems. Even our dogs and cats, the animals we in turn feed, have started to experience the same condition that only humans suffer from. We unfortunately created this by feeding them processed food.

When we were doing anatomy classes in graduate school, we'd often look at the intestinal lining of corpses. Slightly gruesome, I know, but very enlightening. What we saw was intestinal lining - which is supposed to be paper-thin—being ¼ inch thick in humans from bad diets. When food is put in your mouth, it's supposed to be absorbed through this paper thin intestinal lining into the blood stream which then decides what to do with it; but how is that possible when the lining is so thick? When I remember those autopsies it seems amazing that food was actually absorbed through something that thick at all! And as we get older, that lining only gets thicker and thicker because of bad food sources and unhealthy living.

In turn, the body gets less healthy as it needs more food in order to get the nutrients. For example, if our body is craving magnesium, we eat the food that has magnesium in it but our body doesn't absorb it very well. It's the same as someone craving chocolate; really, they're craving the magnesium in the chocolate, but again the body isn't absorbing it. And what happens when we don't absorb the nutrients we need? We eat more! When a person doesn't get the minerals he needs, he continues to eat in order to attain this particular mineral or vitamin that's deficient in the body.

That's a huge cause of overeating. It's our body telling us it needs more.

Think back to what we know about society a few thousand years ago, before cooking began. They didn't have microwaves or all the tools we have today; they didn't have processed milk, fast food or TV dinners. They didn't have apples that would last for months or freezers to store food in for months. They ate what nature gave them; the food God had already cooked for them on the tree. In two thousand years our bodies haven't actually changed much, but our food has altered dramatically.

Being overweight is not the result of having one bad meal. It happens as a result of many bad meals. We can eat tomatoes all year round, or enjoy mangoes no matter where in the world they are grown; it's great to have choice, but what has to be done to our food in order for this to happen? And is that why tomatoes nowadays don't even have half the vitamins they used to 20 to 30 years ago?

Of course, our food should contain all the vitamins we need but with fewer people eating food straight out of the ground, that's becoming harder and harder to achieve. Add to that the fact that our bodies are struggling to absorb what vitamins are there in the first place, and you can see why we need to eat and eat in order to gain enough nutrients to keep our internal engines going. Note what I said there—we crave nutrients, *not* calories. Calories do not fulfill the body by itself; nutrients do.

Picture your body like a car. Ideally, your car would run on diesel and be at its peak efficiency. You live in a remote area, however, where diesel just isn't available; instead, there's the next best thing—diesel light. Ok, so you have to make do with that. The only problem is that where you could 50 miles to the gallon with diesel, you only get 25 with diesel light. To run your car, do your errands and keep up with the demands of your life, you find you need to fill your tank with twice as much fuel as before. And there's another problem. Diesel light contains impurities; additives that enable it to last much longer than ordinary diesel but these 'added extras' start to clog up your filter. This means that over time, less and less of the diesel light is getting to your engine. Your car starts to run sluggishly, and needs more and more diesel light to keep running, as it just isn't capable of using it efficiently. It isn't long before you have to make regular trips to the mechanics yard.

The handy thing about cars, of course, is that you can trade in and trade upwards for a new car whenever you want. You can't do that with your body! It's the body you're born with and it'll be the same body you die with—how soon depends on your decisions!

Why do we eat meals three times a day?

I'll tell you something else as well; years ago, when people didn't have 7-Elevens and 24 hour supermarkets and restaurants, they'd have gaps between their meals. Before harvesting and crops, we'd walk from place to place finding berries and vegetables and eating whatever we found wherever we found it; there would be gaps between food, sometimes even days. Step into modern society and suddenly we're eating three square meals a day 365 days a year and being told it's the right thing. Why? Our bodies haven't changed that much. No other animal eats three times a day aside from humans. Some even hibernate and don't eat anything for weeks. Sometimes fish don't eat for a couple of days. People wonder why we have problems! Killing the goose for the golden egg!

Humans are the only animals to have introduced food-related rituals as well. Who said we should eat Turkey and our entire bodyweight in one sitting at Thanksgiving? We did. The same for birthday or holiday parties; it's almost impossible to eat the right food, isn't it? And imagine going to a barbeque and saying you didn't want a hamburger? It's almost unheard of because we tell ourselves this is what we should be doing, whether our bodies want or need it.

The plain fact is that overeating is just not good for you. People who eat less do a lot better. When researchers look at longevity, they see that people who eat little—they have smaller meals and don't overeat - live longer. That's because their body is actually using the food they are putting into their body and doesn't have to use any extra energy to break down the food it isn't.

Let's address the real issue - ourselves.

Culturally, when a woman looks at the mirror, she thinks she is obese even if she is the thinnest woman in the whole world. On the other hand when an overweight guy looks in the mirror, he thinks he has a six pack and so forth. Beauty really is in eye of the beholder!

All parts of the body, including the brain, are involved in absorbing nutrients. And when that absorption is not as good as it should be, hey, guess what? People are putting on weight and developing heart problems and health.

You could say that we are our own worst enemy; we are creating problems for ourselves. Times have changed significantly and as a result of this, we've created a lot of manmade illnesses. It's reaching a real epidemic and we've seen health care cost soaring as a result of that. We even have people stapling their stomachs because they can't stop themselves from eating too much—who would have thought that would become common place 20 years ago?

Of course, procedures such as stomach stapling are not addressing the real issue at all. These people still have the same brain which tells them how much food to eat; that doesn't change because your stomach is smaller. Their brain will now tell them to eat more than their new stomach can handle, which is why some of them end up in the emergency room. They also still have the same *gastric emptying* rate which is the amount of food that goes through the body before the body signals that it's hungry again.

No, to examine the real underlying problems you need to look at the whole body. That's what chiropractic does. When we look at how the body absorbs nutrients; it involves various different areas of the body. Sometimes it involves the brain, as I've mentioned; there's a reason we talk about comfort eating and a reason people feel compelled to eat more and more—it's their brain telling them they need to.

Sometimes it affects the thyroid, or the nerves in the middle of the neck affect the thyroid; the bones press on the nerves which in turn interfere with proper thyroid function. That thyroid gland may only weigh one ounce but it's an incredibly important part of the body; it secretes hormones that literally tell specific body parts what to do. It controls heat regulation, body temperature and helps the body make more energy, alongside other equally crucial jobs. If your thyroid is out of whack, your body is going to have problems. If this little gland isn't working correctly, people will have a hard time losing weight no matter what diet they're on. That's why in a chiropractic examination we look in the center of the neck to see if the bone protecting the nerve going to the thyroid is affected and try to correct it with a specific chiropractic spinal adjustment. Nerves in the mid-back go to the stomach—these help absorb vitamins and minerals. The nerves in the low back go to the intestines which will help absorbing nutrients and use calories from food.

Five steps to weight loss:

It's easy to list all of the reasons why we've shot ourselves in the foot over recent years, but technology isn't going to go away. Time is still passing. So, how do we get our bodies back on an even keel? How do we undo years of unnatural eating; what can we do to give our bodies the best chance of running on the very best 'diesel' our world has to offer…?

- First, the big one: **STOP DIETING!**

  Dieting won't work; it's not enough. Dieting is an unhealthy person's attempt to change just one thing in their life, to 'become' healthy. But it takes a healthy person to become healthy. You need to change your entire lifestyle instead; it's not enough to just cut out some food or plan to lose 10 pounds—you'll only put the weight back on anyway because the unhealthy practices are still there underneath. Change your eating habits entirely; exercise, do chiropractic care… take steps to change your entire life. Your weight will solve itself if you do that. No one can stick to these crazy diets forever. Once you go on a diet, your body will do anything it can to cling onto the weight you're trying to lose in order to conserve energy. Your own body is fighting you—that should tell you something. A sick minded person who decides to eat healthy will only do so for days to months. A healthy minded person will do it for a lifetime … this is the way to go for success.

- **Avoid sugar content**

  We all know to avoid sugar when we're trying to lose weight, but did you know artificial sweetener can be just as bad for you? I know, I know, you thought it was the healthier option; there's so much confusing advice out there that many people fall for this. But what you're actually doing here is telling the body to expect sugar. The body gets ready for it and releases the same hormones, but you don't actually give it the sugar to use. It isn't healthy; nature didn't create sugar that way. If you can't find an artificial sweetener tree, it can't be right for you!

- **Add muscle mass**

  One of the best things you can do for your body is to build up your muscles; don't worry about looking like a bodybuilder—it's virtually impossible for a lay person to achieve that look. Muscle in the body is a functional metabolic organ which actually controls that way the body functions; when you have more muscles you actually have a better metabolic rate.

  Resistance training weight helps bone density as well; it's the easiest way to strengthen your bones, much more effective than upping your calcium intake. It's a key step to take but, like ditching the diet and changing your lifestyle above, it's going to take time. It's not a quick fix solution; it's a process. It's like growing a tomato plant. You don't plant a seed and the next day a tomato grows.

- **Stop the discomfort**

  Pain stops you from losing weight; you can't exercise and you lose the ability to function normally. Chiropractic can help the body to function better, to check if the organs are working, as well as the thyroid. We can even test if the correct nerve flow is going to the intestines so that it can absorb the vitamins and minerals to get out of pain and heal correctly.

It's important to take the time to make sure your spine is aligned because your nervous system and your spine control all the organs and systems of your body. Without *that* being aligned, you don't have a chance of gaining health.

- **Eat things that aren't cooked**

The more natural foods you eat from better sources. Avoid processed foods since those are better for your body. Eat things that are grown locally and don't have to be transported halfway across the country. Opt for herbs that can make your food taste great *and* help your body function at the same time. Dandelion root, for instance, helps a lot with liver function.

What did we do before tools? If we didn't have the tools to kill chickens or cows, what did we do? We ate fruits and vegetables; crops and harvesting came much later in time. Nowadays we're eating foods that we wouldn't naturally eat if we hadn't invented technology; we would be eating roots and berries instead and everything would be raw. Try it and see how much better you feel.

Signs that the food you're eating is wrong

- **You're tired after food**

We've all done it; eaten a big meal and then fallen asleep shortly after. You probably didn't think anything of it, but in actual fact, that's a problem. Eating the wrong food, or too much of it, shows symptoms and if you eat food and then *lose* energy, that's not good! Our body is like a sponge; it can only absorb so much—it has to do *something* with the extra food. That's when the body then works overtime to put the food somewhere, usually converting it directly into fat. So you've created fat and tired yourself out at the same time! How can that be a good thing?

- **You wouldn't find it in nature**

  I've mentioned this before with the sweetener tree above, but I think it's worth making the point again. We can buy all sorts of crazy food these days, some we now take for granted and don't even think twice about. They mix cow's milk with strawberries to make a milkshake, for instance—that's kind of peculiar! Where do cow's milk and strawberries show up together in nature? They don't. I doubt cows would even eat strawberries if they had the chance, as delicious as they can be. We also hear all this talk about taking 'natural vitamins'—really, natural? Where can you *find* a vitamin tree?

  And that's a good rule of thumb for your food intake—if it's synthetic and designed or created by man and not nature, it isn't healthy. Keep reminding yourself of that. Also if you can't pronounce it, it's probably not good for you. Food is simple. That item you buy in the store has more than 10 ingredients be will confusing to your body. It's got to figure out what to do with all the different ingredients. Let's think how in natural a peanut which grows in the ground would mix itself with a grape?

- **You're only taking out and not adding to your system**

  I tell my patients that I don't recommend alcohol intake, but I also tell them it's a balancing act; if you do drink alcohol, you need to do something to handle the poison you're putting into your body. So you should drink extra water or have some fruit after an alcoholic beverage in order to replenish the body. If you drink alcohol, you're just taking vitamins away from the body and not adding anything to it, so you need to concentrate on putting some more vitamins into your system.

  How best to do that? How can you be sure that what you buy or eat avoids artificial flavors and colors? The most obvious way is to grow it yourself. That way you know exactly what has gone into and onto your food before it hits your plate. If that isn't an option for you, buy from a local farm, or from an organic supermarket. In fact, let's look at the order in which you should consume your food to be as healthy as possible:

1. First choice: Grow your own
2. Second choice: Buy from a local organic farm
3. Third choice: Buy organic from a great store
4. Fourth choice: Buy organic from a regular store
4. Fifth choice: Buy regular food
6. Sixth choice: Buy canned/ frozen food
7. Seventh choice: Buy processed foods.

This is a good list to live by. If you can mostly stay at the top of this list, you're onto a winner!

Chapter 12

How to Give Your Child the Best Start in Life

We have talked about the spine individually and we have a choice to call a chiropractor and get checked for misalignment, but what about those who can't use the phone? I'm going to say something that will probably shock you right now; as we discussed earlier, our bodies are meant to heal themselves but sometimes stress gets in the way. That applies to children as well as adults. A child born ill will do everything it can to get healthy, while a child born healthy will actually *find* a way to become ill through bad diet and lifestyle.

I know, it sounds crazy but it's true. We see it every day. That's why I tell people that children can benefit from chiropractic too.

Perhaps the best proof of my conviction is whether I would treat my own child with chiropractic. And yes, my son got his first adjustment at only 6 minutes old (the first 5 minutes I was so amazed I actually forgot). When you learn that you are going to be a father for the first time, it is humbling; knowing that you will be responsible for someone so tiny and helpless is overwhelming. Think about it—they can't move, they can't talk; when things bother or upset them they can't communicate that besides a cry, which could mean anything! They can't make their own money, get their own food or drive to the store! It's pretty stressful! I compare it to a person who is tied up in a straight jacket in another country who can't speak the language and has a fly buzzing around their nose. Not a very enjoyable time.

You want to change the world for them, make it a better place so nothing can ever hurt them; hold them close and promise them that you will do everything within your power to protect them.

Our power is limited. What you can do, however, is use whatever knowledge you have to ensure they get the very best start in life.

It also means that I will use chiropractic to make sure he never develops the problems that plague so many adults. From the second he is born, in fact even before that point, I will give him the best chance at health that I can. Other parents can do it too.

Indeed, my wife got adjusted at regular points throughout her pregnancy and she loved it; she was convinced it made the pregnancy easier for her and my son. And do you know what else? From the back, she didn't even look as though she was pregnant. It was amazing! But from the side she just looked like she'd swallowed a basketball!

Chiropractic helped her feel more confident about our son's health, and it's important to let people know that it can do the same for their children too. The chiropractic approach to children's health is very different from the mainstream so I'm going to take some time to explain what we know about birth and bringing up a child and how you can use nature's principles to strengthen their body before they are even born!

Let me elaborate on what I said earlier. My experience has been, especially with children, that when a sick child is born it actually does whatever it can to be healthy. That's a credit to the healer inside all of us.

Unfortunately, children who are born healthy do whatever they can to become sick. It's true. They eat the wrong food, they don't exercise and basically they take health for granted. A little like a lot of adults!

Modern society and medicine today is moving us away from nature; the very way children are brought up has changed dramatically since we developed all this technology that allows children to sit around indoors for hours on end and never get any exercise.

When I was a child, I would have hated the thought of an entire day spent inside; if it rained, I used to go crazy because I wanted to be out, running about and playing with my friends. This is when video games weren't as sophisticated. And that wasn't all that long ago! Nowadays, however, children play with their friends remotely; they meet them in chat rooms, in video games and on instant messenger. They spend hours talking without even getting any fresh air.

When they do surface from their rooms, they eat food that hasn't seen a field in days; it's been frozen, processed and changed beyond all recognition. In between meals, they snack on potato chips and candy, rather than an apple or a banana.

When they inevitably become ill because their immune system has been deprived of the nutrients it needs to stay strong, the medical community tries to cure whatever is wrong with them at the time. So if they suffer from headaches, they'll look at the head; if they complain about stomach pains, they'll only look at the stomach. They won't look any further to see what is the underlying problem, or address the very poor lifestyles that our children live nowadays. Really, we're not giving our children a very good start in life, are we?

Chiropractic believes very strongly that we need to get back to nature where our children are concerned. And that we need to do it from before they are even born.

Let's take a look at the birth process. You obviously have the same processes—conception, the admission to the hospital, contraction, dilation, transmission, get the baby crowning, give birth, after birth and discharge from the hospital—but chiropractors handle it differently.

We know that most women nowadays deliver on their backs. They are laid on their backs and the babies are delivered with the help of forceps or pulling. *Why is pulling needed?* Because the child has to go against gravity to be born; when you deliver a child this way, you actually have to pull the baby up out of the mother against gravitational forces.

Women assume that it was always this way, but that's not true. This actually all started way back with a king of France; you won't believe this story, but I'll tell you anyway. You see, the king happened to be a kind of pervert and he wanted to actually see the birth process, even though at this time men were not allowed to see a woman naked. Incredibly, the people who delivered children were actually male barbers; for some reason, these people were paid to commit murders for the government and also do the autopsies and dissections. As a result, the barbers came to know the human body better than the doctors themselves, so they were the ones who delivered children.

Of course, they were men and weren't allowed to actually see the birth, so that made things a little challenging! To get around it, they would tie a cloth around the barber's neck and also around the mother's neck, as they weren't allowed to see her intimate parts. Then they would kind of go back and forth and the babies would be delivered without the barbers seeing anything at all. Ingenious, in its own way!

Anyway, the king of France wanted to see the birth process so he would hide himself and watch. From there it started to become more acceptable for a man to see a woman during childbirth and for the woman to be lying down during it.

So for this reason, women now give birth in a way that completely traumatizes the child. Because you're going against gravity, it takes a lot of pressure to deliver the baby; you are literally pulling the baby out of the womb. This places a lot of pressure on the baby, especially on its head. Imagine it: let's say you went to the mall and I was there with my baby. If I grabbed the baby's head and started dangling it, what would your response be? You'd tell me to stop wouldn't you? And of course, you'd be right. You would feel that I am hurting the child, because everyone knows that the first time you hold a newborn, you protect its head. So, let me ask you this: what's the difference between me dangling a baby by its head, versus a doctor pulling a baby by its head out of the mother's womb? The answer is not much. The pressure that it places on the baby is pretty much the same.

You have to realize how terrifying birth is for a baby; it's very traumatic. It is very easy to damage a baby's nerve system during and after birth, just by the environment that it finds itself in. Let's have a think about what happens when a baby is born. Typically what happens is that when the baby comes out of the mother the very environment shocks their nervous system. It usually goes on a cold scale, for instance—that shocks the baby. You are taking a child from a very dark, warm and secluded area to a bright and very loud room which is a shock. The first thing to do is to get the child's spine checked by a chiropractic who knows how to look for the nervous system and make sure that the spine is working, all this shock is incredible stress. Remember, the nervous system is the most important system! If it started this baby organs', you should take care of it.

So, are there more natural ways to give birth? Remember, natural means less pressure for the child. And yes, there are:

Natural ways to give birth

- **Use gravity**. Don't make the baby fight gravity to be born; it only serves to make childbirth more painful and traumatic. One of the best approaches to deliver a child is a home birth because it's more natural. Walk around, do what you feel you need to do to get this child to be born; it's the one thing they stop you from doing in the hospital. I remember my mother telling me that all she wanted to do when I was being born was to walk about until I was ready to come out; the hospital wouldn't let her. They made her lie on a bed instead. How did that help?

- **Have a water birth**. You have to realize that prior to being born, a baby is more of an amphibian than a mammal because it's living in liquid. So a water birth will instantly make the child feel more comfortable. Basically, in a water birth the child is coming out from liquid into another liquid environment, so it's less distressing. By keeping the temperature of the water as near to maternal temperature as possible, the child notices less of a difference, hence its stress is reduced. The baby then takes its first breath once it is lifted out of the water (only a few moments after being born) and can feel the difference in environment; babies cannot breathe underwater and various factors ensure they do not try to.

Why is this so important?

When a child is being born, the pressure it is subjected to inevitably has an effect on its spine. How can it not? As chiropractors, we specifically look at areas of the spine which will have been affected by the pulling that happens in childbirth. A baby is going to cry if it's hurt but it's also going to cry for several other reasons such as room temperature, hunger etc. So, how do you actually know that there is something wrong with your baby? The baby is not going to tell you 'hey listen; there is something wrong at the top of my spine because I was pulled on. Can you give me over to a chiropractor?'

Now the child grows up and is learning how to walk. Based on studies, a child falls down up to 1,500 times while it's learning how to walk; as it grows up and begins playing with other children; it causes injuries to the spine some more. A child will not know when it has a tiny injury and this, along with other problems, will continue to affect the spine negatively till the child grows up to be a teenager and then he or she may get back problems and go for chiropractic adjustment. As a parent I would think that if I didn't see blood and my son stops crying he is fine—not true!

However, misalignments could happen right from day one when the baby is being pulled from the mother during C-section or natural birth. That's why I think it is so crucial that children are seen by a chiropractor as soon as possible after birth. I wish every person had pain as a young child. They would check early-on problems that were unfixable later on! Close to 40% of my new patients come in with problems that started within the first 6 months of their life! Unfortunately these patients many times are even older than 40 years and never knew these problems were marinating for all that time. Our last spinal checkups usually occurred when we were in grade school.

Chapter 13

Is it Safe to Use Chiropractic on a Child?

Chiropractic adjustment on a child is extremely safe. Imagine closing your eyes and putting your finger against an eyeball. The amount of pressure you feel on your eyeball is exactly the amount we would adjust a child with. My experience has been that the kids of chiropractors were very upset with the fact that they didn't have a lot of sick days during the school year!

My son got fussy over only a few things—namely food and gas/burping. When he is hungry we would feed him of course; when he is gassy we would burp him. Sometimes, however, he still won't settle; like a lot of parents we've tried numerous things to burp him or stop him crying but they don't always work. However when I do an adjustment it works instantly; a burp that doesn't come up now comes up, a cry that won't go away is now gone. It's very interesting. As time went one he would just get close to the special equipment I used to adjust him and he would stop crying instantly and I haven't even treated him yet. He develops lean and muscular and outgrew all of his age group's clothes.

I spoke to another chiropractor whose child was born only a few weeks before and he notices that his girl is having the same responses; when I see other patient's children I notice a difference but when it's yours it's a miracle! My wife says to me quite regularly: "Thank god I married a chiropractor!"

You see children that are seen by a chiropractor tend to be healthier and also, as babies, they did not get vaccinated. I'll come onto the vaccination issue in a little while. On the whole, they tend to live a healthier lifestyle; so many illnesses are bypassed as a result of a proper spine. When my sister-in-law was delivering my niece I ran to the hospital and adjusted my niece who was only 3 hours old at that time. Children respond so well to chiropractic adjustments! They sometimes start giggling and it's amazing!

We don't twist the neck or anything, so it is perfectly safe.

You can change the type of spine adjustment needed depending on the child.

There are two particular methods you can adjust a child with. One is at the top of the spine and the other is at the bottom of the spine. As chiropractors we look for these areas because they tend to be the areas that cause the most problems. Misalignment at the top of the spine happens because a child has this big heavy head and very little muscles on the neck and a lot a problems show up that way.

The other method is to adjust the bottom of the spine because they are sitting on it and falling on it every now and then as they're trying to crawl and move. These two particular methods in chiropractic are very effective. The adjustments at the top of the neck are geared for a child who has a lot of ear infections and gets a lot of colds. The adjustments at the bottom of the spine adjust the whole spine to help the baby relax better; it also affects colic and digestive problems.

First, typically, they are taken back by someone not their parents touching the spine. On their first adjustment it's usually a fight and they're crying, but after their first adjustment they run up as fast as they can to be the first to get a treatment. It's great to deliver health care that is safe, all natural, and feels really great. Chiropractors who work with children know what to look for. There are curves that have to develop in the spine, for instance, as a sign of proper development. One of the first things you look for is a curve in the neck. This tends to happen as the baby is learning to crawl and it's lifting its head up in order to look forward. If this curve didn't happen, your baby would not be developing well.

This curve is instrumental in supporting the rest of the spine to make the development that it needs for progress. One of the other curves you are looking for is the low back curve which happens as a result of sitting and them trying to learn how to walk and crawl. This is very instrumental later in their development. If these changes do not develop correctly, you can see it later in patients in their 20s or 30s. There is an old saying that goes 'as you bend the twig so grows the tree'. You take a child and you bend the twig the wrong way and the tree (i.e. when the child grows up to an adult) bends the wrong way as well.

If a child has this spinal misalignment at the top of the spine for too long, for instance, it can result in arthritis which is inflexible. You have to do a chiropractic test to detect this. You are just not going to get that done by a pediatrician or any other medical examination. The chiropractor you are using must be certified and familiar with how to treat children. That's very important because not all chiropractors are familiar with this.

As I mentioned in an earlier chapter, I use the Pierce Results system of chiropractic. This method is very scientific. It has specific strategies for fixing a person's spine and improving his or her health. When we take a patient under care, we're really looking to pin point exactly what's causing this person to become sick. *Unlike traditional medicine!*

> ### *EXAMPLE*
>
> *Here's an example of how chiropractic can be SUCCESSFULLY used on children:*
>
> *We see a lot of little kids, two to three years old, with horrible earaches. These come from one particular bone in the spine that has moved in a particular way; when you spot it, it's clear as day. There's nothing worse than earache; for such a relatively minor issue, it can be incredibly painful. Children do fantastic after this adjustment and believe it or not, they respond better than adults. That's obviously because their bodies are still developing. They find that they don't have earache anymore and I can't tell you how happy they—and their parents—feel afterwards!*

The Pierce Results System uses three ways of adjusting the spine, which are unlike any other method in chiropractic. It works very well for children. For instance:

- There is a *segmental* approach to the spine which simply means going vertebrae by vertebrae and putting them back in place very specifically. This is a traditional way of adjusting the spine that most chiropractors use—the way they do it is different but the purpose is the same. This is like the trees, this fixes the bigger dents.

- There is also a *tonal* way of adjusting the spine. Tonal approach is about getting the nervous system, the major component within the spine, and the spinal cords to relax so that they can function at a higher level—think of it as upgrading your "health" system. If everything is in order, it's much easier to heal! This is like fertilizing a tree in the forest. This is the fine tuning.

- The next approach is *global* in which the entire body is properly aligned. You're not just looking at how one bone sits next to another bone but you're looking instead at the entire picture and putting it back in the right perspective. You can see this with balance, coordination and posture. This is the whole forest alignment. It's like all trees lined up in a row.

All three of these are very important for a child's development.

The *segmental* approach is needed because of birth trauma; *tonal,* because the baby is developing its nervous system very quick and *global* because the child has to stand up straight and strong. All three have a hand in how the baby develops and whether the child can bypass a lot of childhood problems as a result of chiropractic care. All these tests are not performed elsewhere in healthcare.

Should you give Your Child Vaccines?

I said I'd come back to this, so let's talk vaccines. As a father, I have strong opinions on vaccines; this is another example of how my views differ from traditional medicine. I believe vaccines can have their place, but I do question it. Let's consider that a baby does not have a strong immune system before it's about six months old. It gains its immune system through its mother's milk; it's amazing, isn't it, just how much nature has taken care of? Anyway, the only protective barrier this baby has is its skin. So what do we do? We give it a chemical vaccine that injects toxic chemicals past the skin. Not just once, or twice, or even within single figures. Within the first six months, a child is given 45 different vaccines. Yes, you read that right: 45! In my eyes, 45 strong chemicals to one weak undeveloped immune system baby is not good!

By the time they are 18 months old they get 64 vaccines and by 46 months they get up to 74 vaccines injected into the body. That's a conservative estimate considering the fact that there are actually 200 vaccines in development.

Let's also consider that vaccines are given based on a germ theory—the theory that all contagious diseases are caused by microorganisms - not germ fact, germ theory. Germs are thought to make someone sick so as a society we attack them with drugs, antibacterial soap etc... However that should only be really true if germs were present in very high concentrations for a HEALTHY person with a good immune system.

The problem is that with this hygiene, we have destroyed our immune systems so much that we are now subject to sickness from even microscopic germs 1/millionth of our body weight.

Vaccine strains are actually not the major problem with vaccines. So why are vaccines bad? Well, let's see. Aside from the fact that most of these vaccines have never been proved to be needed, much less safe, let's take a moment to look at what is actually inside these vaccines:

- *Latex rubber* - which is life threatening

- *MSG* (the thing you try to avoid in Chinese restaurants) - this is a nerve toxin which is quite allergenic

- *Aluminum*—which not only affects the baby's ability to heal correctly but increases the chances of having Alzheimer's disease later in life

- *Formaldehyde*—which is carcinogenic, namely causes cancer. This is what they put in dead people in order to preserve them! I remember in graduate school when we did autopsies, they would fill the room with this toxic smell—many people were allergic to it. If this preserves a dead body for months it doesn't belong in a live one.

- *Phenol*—phenol is anti-freeze—truly! This is what you'd normally use in your car! And not surprisingly, it affects a baby's immune system and health adversely

- *Mercury*—which is poisonous and can damage the nerves; it has also been linked to autism. It's amazing that mercury is not allowed in any dosage in fish or even a household thermometer but is still allowed in a vaccine for humans. Why?

These things are all used to stabilize the active ingredients in the vaccines. The problem is that they are highly toxic and dangerous to the body.

Did you know, for instance, that when a baby screams as it is given a vaccination, it isn't always because of the shock of a needle prick; it can also be a result of minor brain damage? It's obviously a very controversial topic; all this is documented and you can find it online. Parents should research this; don't just take my word for it. There is great research available out there and also a website www.909shot.com that can give you information on this.

The medical profession tells us that our children should have vaccinations; that we are failing our children if we do not. They don't like people who question it; they try to enforce it at every step.

They won't even allow your child to go to school if they're not vaccinated. What harm will my kid do to all the kids that are vaccinated? If they're already vaccinated against all the diseases! They won't get it since they are so 'safe' how could they give it to my son? That's the sort of contrary idea that surrounds the issue of vaccinations.

I guess as a parent, you have to set the example; I know that my child will not be vaccinated. There are too many unknowns;

no one has really proved these vaccines are safe—and they are certainly not natural. The debate about autism and vaccines, for instance, still has not been resolved to my satisfaction.

I have child patients who were normal before they were vaccinated and then got unexpected problems show up. Who knows if they would have shown up anyway but it's certainly a coincidence isn't it? Too many coincidences in my opinion! The natural argument given by medical doctors is that autism happens to a very low percentage of kids. Would you play Russian roulette with your child? How do we know that a life-threatening disease or even cancer that is triggered later in life wasn't given to him as a child by vaccination? Do we know the absolute cause of cancer?

Additionally, if people aren't sick who do you sell the drugs to?

There are just too many questions. And as a parent you have to do what you think is best for your child. That's why my child will not have any vaccines but will certainly have chiropractic to make sure he is healthy, from birth onwards.

'Health is not the absence of disease, anymore than wealth is an absence of poverty'

I am dedicated to giving him the very best start in life, just like all good parents do.

Chapter 14

How You Can See Success in Your Spine

When we make a chiropractic adjustment we can see all sorts of results, some immediate, some developing over time, within the entire body. Small adjustments can correct and alter posture, improve movement, aid balance and increase strength.

The opposite is also true. If we do not receive chiropractic treatment and let our bones, joints and muscles do as they will, we can also contribute to a loss of balance, poor joint movement as our joints start to seize and pain caused by poor posture.

So let's take a look at each of the above in more detail.

Posture

When we talk about posture, most people think we're talking about simply sitting and standing up straight. They picture young women in finishing school with books on their heads, trying to learn the best way to stand tall.

Let's not underplay it, however. Poor posture has far reaching consequences for the health of our bodies.

The human body needs alignment. Ideally, our bones stack on top of one another; the head rests directly on top of the spine, which sits on top of our shoulders, which sits directly over the pelvis and hips, which sits over the knees and ankles. This helps to ensure that our bones—and not our muscles—support our weight.

It is easy to interfere with this delicate balance, however. If you spend hours every day sitting in a chair, or hunching forward or doing any of the things that put unwanted pressure on your joints such as balancing your weight primarily on one leg, it causes chronic muscle tension.

That's because your muscles in the neck and back have to carry the weight of the body; it means your spine is no longer supporting your body the way that it should.

This chronic tension and resulting joint pressure leads to shoulder and back pain, as well as headaches; add to that depression and problems with your attention span and the problems start to stack up.

Yes, posture ranks right there; it's as crucial as healthy eating, exercising and getting enough sleep. A good posture empowers everything you do in your life; it gives you energy, helps you feel healthier and enables you to move gracefully. If you lack good posture, you can actually damage your spine every time you exercise; it's near impossible to be fully physically fit.

So, what can you do if you already have bad posture?

- Eliminate 'bad stress' from your body. It could be a poorly adjusted workstation at work, a purse that's too heavy, high heels, big wallet or anything else that causes your body to move away from its center.

- Just as you remove bad stress from your body, so should you apply 'good stress' to it. Exercise, stretches, spinal adjustments and changes to your environment are important ways to regain your center of balance.

Movement

You heard the story of Barbara Pollard's frozen shoulder and partial paralysis direct from her husband's mouth. Reverend Pollard told us that his wife couldn't even lift her arms up above her head.

Imagine if that happened to you. If one morning you woke with a frozen shoulder and you couldn't move your upper arm more than a few inches in any direction.

That could cause considerable inconvenience, if not outright pain. You wouldn't be able to drive a car, do your work; you wouldn't even be able to dress yourself!

What's more, just how much would you be able to concentrate on *anything* other than the problems with your arm?

It's the same with any part of your body; if any part of your body isn't moving the way it is supposed to, it will cause problems with your everyday life.

So, just what happens when people experience back pain, for instance? Many patients report that they were doing something relatively benign—putting out the milk bottles, bending to pick up the newspaper—when they felt sudden pain. Obviously our bodies shouldn't react so dramatically to something so simple, but there must be a problem already, right?

Picture the joints in your body being 'locked up'—it's a little like severe rust on an object that over time starts to impact on the movement of the hinges. The same is true of the body; joints can end up barely moving at all. When this happens, other areas of the body are forced to move in order to compensate.

Imagine the stress on these other joints; it's no wonder it soon starts to feel painful and suffer from inflammation. It's like hurting your leg; even if you use crutches, you are forced to put more stress and strain on the remaining healthy leg until that too starts to feel painful.

And now those areas that first had a problem slowly start to worsen as the muscles continue to tighten, joints stick together and ligaments and tendons shorten. If this is not addressed, it's no wonder even the slightest motion can cause painful episodes at the smallest movement.

Imagine an elderly person who can't walk well; you can almost see their body seizing up before your eyes. Despite common perception, this isn't an inevitable result of aging; instead it's a consequence of not keeping the body mobile via exercise and healthy alignment.

Stretching can help maintain mobility, as can regular chiropractic adjustments.

Why is this so important? As well as maintaining movement as I mentioned before, keeping the body supple is a good defense against pain and disability.

Strength

Picture your muscles as the wires that hold up a radio or television antenna. If the wires are equally strong on all sides, the antenna will stand up straight. So will you! Your muscles are a key to keeping your body upright and allowing you to move.

If those antenna wires break or become weak on one side, however, the antenna will lean or collapse. Again, so will your body!

Muscles become strong or weak depending on what you ask them to do; do plenty of exercise and your muscles in the affected areas will be stronger. Live a sedentary lifestyle and your muscles will be weaker.

That said, those muscles you do use everyday—even in normal everyday living such as sitting at a desk all day ('exercising' the muscles in the upper back and chest)—will become stronger.

Sitting at a desk all day may help certain muscles, but it won't help the muscles at the back; this imbalance can lead to chronic muscle spasms.

And what happens then? You're lopsided! Ok, maybe not literally, but the imbalance of muscles can contribute to poor posture in your spine. And you already know the consequences of that.

Left unchecked, muscle imbalances tend to get worse, not better.

The easiest way to correct this imbalance is with specific exercises to develop the back muscles and chiropractic care. Once the muscles in your middle back are strong, the poor posture improves.

Balance

Without balance, life is one long tightrope.

Balance exists when muscle coordination is encouraged. Exercises such as walking, swimming, yoga, Pilates, bicycling, martial arts and bodybuilding all help to improve muscle coordination and therefore balance.

On the opposite side, sedentary activities such as watching television, reading and working at a desk (that problem again!) not surprisingly do the opposite.

It is easy to have extreme stress in the muscles as a result of sitting for many hours every day without exercising. This tension contributes to restricted movement and joint pain if it is not addressed.

All of the above should hopefully help you realize just how important it is to pay attention to your spine. Treat it well, and treat it often. Think of a regular visit to your chiropractor as you do the six monthly check ups to your dentist or a health checkup with your doctor. Make it an important part of your health routine.

It really can mean the difference between a life half lived with aches, pains and illnesses, or a life free to stretch, breathe deeply and enjoy the wonderful things that life offers. Think of it for yourself, your partner and your children. Your knowledge is not power, it's the use of knowledge that is power.

Take to heart the advice I've given you and try to get back to basics; live as we used to live, with fresh healthy fruit and vegetables, regular exercise and a positive spirit. Try to tone down the unhealthy additions that technology has brought us as much as you can.

I hope this book in its entirety will inspire and encourage you to change your life for the better, to actively seek out and follow good health.

I wish you health and happiness for many years to come!

About the Author

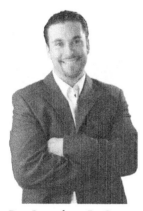

Dr. Jonathan B. Spages

Dr. Jonathan Spages is a name that conjures up countless personalities. An active social worker, loving husband, doting father, published author, dynamic presenter and teacher , but most of all, a man who has a passion for health, fitness and a keen sense of wellness.

He is highly qualified in the latest technique called the Pierce Results System for spinal correction, and has a successful practice in New Jersey.

Dr. Spages is a talented speaker and presenter, and his positive, clear-cut, and motivational approach has earned him rave reviews and a huge fan following. He is frequently interviewed, giving a number of radio and television addresses on a wide range of health topics.

In the course of his career, Dr. Spages has won many awards and scaled new heights. He continues to add to his impressive portfolio and in addition has been named a U.S. Chamber of Commerce Wellness Coach in 2009 and was given a Best Business Practices in Paterson award that same year. His contribution to charity and social work is second to none and he has assisted in a number of events including a mission trip to El Salvador, a cultural study in Thailand and sponsorship of Kids Day America from 2003 through 2005.

Dr. Spages has been privileged to help the workers of 911 and also actively been involved with professional athletes.

Special Offer!

Valuable health information that will change your life, a special gift for The Wellness Approach Readers!

Here's what you'll get:

- Dr. Spages powerful audio interview CD. Hear the ture story about how chiropractic saved his father's life. This CD is packed with valuable health information and breakthrough never know before and advice, everything you need to get healthy right away!

- Dr Spages' Private Health Newsletter.

  This newsletter is full of cutting edge studies and information that will help guide you to the best health decisions.

- Dr. Spages' exclusive book "101 Unique Ways to Get Healthy!". This book is packed with information you wont find somewhere else. Dr. Spages tells it all in this simple book. A must for health nuts!

Ready to get your free book and gifts?
Come visit us at:
WWW.THEWELLNESSAPPROACHBOOK.COM
To grab yours today!

DON'T JUST TAKE MY WORD FOR IT...

In 1928, a medical doctor called Dr. Windsor tried to prove that chiropractic DIDN'T work. He just couldn't believe that a patient could have a spinal adjustment and see improvements in their organs.

He dissected 22 human and cat cadavers. And what did he find?

- 96 percent of the 220 organs he looked at were a result of a bone being out of place
- The 21 heart cases Dr. Windsor looked at had misaligned bones at the top of their necks.
- All 17 cases of kidney-related deaths had misaligned bones at their lower backs.
- He had no choice but to directly correlate organ function to the spine.

Chiropractic Science Proven beyond a doubt!

BUY A SHARE OF THE FUTURE IN YOUR COMMUNITY

These certificates make great holiday, graduation and birthday gifts that can be personalized with the recipient's name. The cost of one S.H.A.R.E. or one square foot is $54.17. The personalized certificate is suitable for framing and will state the number of shares purchased and the amount of each share, as well as the recipient's name. The home that you participate in "building" will last for many years and will continue to grow in value.

Here is a sample SHARE certificate:

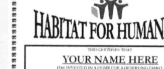

HABITAT FOR HUMANITY

THIS CERTIFIES THAT
YOUR NAME HERE
HAS INVESTED IN A HOME FOR A DESERVING FAMILY

1985-2005
TWENTY YEARS OF BUILDING FUTURES IN OUR
COMMUNITY ONE HOME AT A TIME

1200 SQUARE FOOT HOUSE @ $65,000 = $54.17 PER SQUARE FOOT
This certificate represents a tax deductible donation. It has no cash value.

YES, I WOULD LIKE TO HELP!

I support the work that Habitat for Humanity does and I want to be part of the excitement! As a donor, I will receive periodic updates on your construction activities but, more importantly, I know my gift will help a family in our community realize the dream of homeownership. **I would like to SHARE in your efforts against substandard housing in my community!** *(Please print below)*

PLEASE SEND ME _____ SHARES at $54.17 EACH = $ $_____

In Honor Of: _____

Occasion: (Circle One)   HOLIDAY   BIRTHDAY   ANNIVERSARY

OTHER: _____

Address of Recipient: _____

Gift From: _____ *Donor Address:* _____

Donor Email: _____

I AM ENCLOSING A CHECK FOR $ $_____ PAYABLE TO HABITAT FOR HUMANITY OR PLEASE CHARGE MY VISA OR MASTERCARD *(CIRCLE ONE)*

Card Number _____ Expiration Date: _____

Name as it appears on Credit Card _____ Charge Amount $ _____

Signature _____

Billing Address _____

Telephone # Day _____ Eve _____

PLEASE NOTE: Your contribution is tax-deductible to the fullest extent allowed by law.
Habitat for Humanity • P.O. Box 1443 • Newport News, VA 23601 • 757-596-5553
www.HelpHabitatforHumanity.org

CPSIA information can be obtained
at www.ICGtesting.com
Printed in the USA
BVOW08s1342310317
479835BV00001B/2/P